The Sprouting Book

Ann Wigmore

AVERY
a member of Penguin Putnam Inc.

The therapeutic procedures in this book are based on the training, personal experiences, and research of the author. Because each person and situation are unique, the author and publisher urge the reader to check with a qualified health professional before using any procedure where there is any question as to its appropriateness.

The publisher does not advocate the use of any particular diet and health program, but believes the information presented in this book should be available to the public.

Because there is always some risk involved, the author and publisher are not responsible for any adverse effects or consequences resulting from the use of any of the suggestions, preparations, or procedures in this book. Please do not use the book if you are unwilling to assume the risk. Feel free to consult a physician or other qualified health professional. It is a sign of wisdom, not cowardice, to seek a second or third opinion.

Cover design by Rudy Shur and Martin Hochberg
Cover photo by Martin Hochberg
In-house editor Diana Puglisi

Library of Congress Cataloging-in-Publication Data

Wigmore, Ann, 1909–
    The sprouting book.

    Includes index.
    1. Cookery (Sprouts)   2. Sprouts.   3. Raw food
diet.   I. Title.
TX801.W49   1986   641.6'5   86–10713
ISBN   0-89529-246-7   (pbk.)

Printed in the United States of America

40 39 38 37

Contents

Preface

Sprouts, while inexpensive and easy to grow, afford one of the most concentrated but truly natural sources of vitamins, minerals, enzymes, and amino acids (protein) known. They are also *biogenic*—alive—and capable of transferring their life energy to your body.

Biogenic foods are foods that when planted will create new life. All raw, unsprouted seeds, beans, grains, and nuts are biogenic. When they are sprouted and eaten, they provide the body with a form of living energy—a composite of vital food factors not yet isolated by scientists, but proven to be of value in nature's laboratory of day-to-day life.

Other important foods, such as fresh vegetables and fruits (before cooking), are considered *bioactive*. That is, while they are rich in organic vitamins, minerals, proteins, and living enzymes, and can contribute to improved well-being, they are not capable of creating new life.

At the other extreme are processed, denatured, and cooked foods, on which I feel modern people have become altogether too dependent. In the Living Food Lifestyle, I suggest that these foods be eaten infrequently or avoided altogether.

Some thirty-five years ago, I began my search for a food or combination of natural ingredients that could regenerate and rejuvenate my own ailing body. For years I had suffered with poor digestion, which finally resulted in colitis, a form of intestinal irritation and bleeding. In addition, arthritis was beginning to stiffen my joints and my hair was turning grey.

I found what I was looking for, and much more—an edible plant food that would grow indoors in any climate and mature in a few days, rather than the 50 to 130 days required to grow fresh fruits and vegetables. An inexpensive food that would rival red meat and garden produce in nutritional value, would need no processing or preparation, and would be easy to digest, even for people with weak digestion. What I found was sprouted seeds, beans, grains, and nuts. (A fuller account of my search for healthful plant foods appears in my autobiography, *Why Suffer?*)

When you eat a sprout you are eating a tiny, easy-to-digest plant that is at its peak of nutritional value. The seed releases all of its stored nutrients in a burst of vitality as it attempts to become a full-sized plant. When you eat a sprout, you literally get the best of what a seed, be it radish, alfalfa, or any of the other edible varieties, has to offer in terms of nutrition.

For more than thirty-five years, I have run a series of two-week educational programs at my health center in Boston, and in lectures around the world, I have taught tens of thousands of people how to control their diet and improve health using my Living Food Diet. This natural foods diet is composed of raw, uncooked foods such as sprouts, greens, fresh vegetables and fruits, sea vegetables, and naturally fermented products. This diet has grown in popularity over the years, and has become the nucleus of a practical form of truly healthful living.

At the very center of the Living Food Diet are sprouts and indoor garden greens. In fact, up to fifty percent of the food served at the Ann Wigmore Foundation consists of fresh sprouts and greens, all grown right on the premises. I myself have lived primarily on sprouted seeds, beans, grains, and nuts for more than two decades. Not only have I healed my body of colitis and arthritis following such a regimen, but I have also achieved a greater level of vitality and health than I had even as a child— and I am no child at seventy-seven. And my hair has returned to its natural brown color, too!

Sprouts are food for a new generation, and for our own *re*generation as well. In *The Sprouting Book*, you will learn the "secrets" of my success growing and using sprouts to improve health.

Chapter 1 begins by tracing the history of sprouts as food through the ages. The second chapter discusses the nutritional value of various sprouts. Chapter 3 focuses on the healing attributes of sprouts. The economics of sprouting are examined on both a personal and a global scale in Chapter 4. Chapters 5 through 8 show you how you can grow and use the best-looking, best-tasting sprouts possible. Chapter 5 lists the different kinds of seeds you can buy for sprouting and offers tips on selecting them. Chapter 6 contains complete instructions for several methods of growing a home sprout garden, and Chapter 7 explains how you can grow salad greens indoors as well.

Chapter 8 features many delicious recipes using sprouts. From the making of crisp flatbreads and filling vegetarian entrees to non-dairy milks and ice creams, you will learn how to use sprouts to dazzle the tastebuds of even fussy eaters, while helping them to better health at the same time. Chapter 9 illustrates two other aspects of the complete sprouting lifestyle: ways of growing sprouts while traveling or camping, and how to use sprouts to improve the health of your pets.

You don't have to be a fanatic to enjoy the flavor and health benefits of sprouts. The addition of even a cup or two of sprouts to your daily diet will make a big difference in the way you feel. Sprouting fits into almost any lifestyle. It is ideal for dieters, growing children, the elderly, vegetarians, athletes, people on the go who don't always eat right, and anyone who wants to look and feel better.

In more ways than one, sprouts are food for a new generation. Aren't you ready for economic savings, renewed health and vigor, and the variety and great taste of sprouts—the unique, life-giving food?

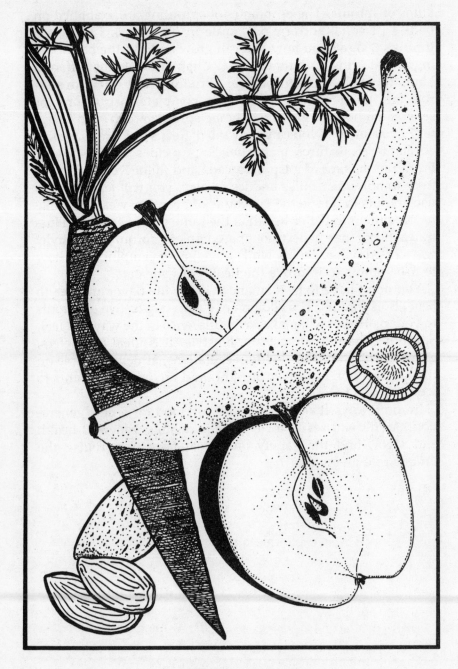

Nutritious Living Foods

1

Ancient Medicine, Modern Food

Germinated and sprouted seeds are instinctive, primeval foods of man, with many millions of years of phylogenetic [evolutionary] affinity.

Edmond Szekely

The history of the various ways sprouts have been used is fascinating. Sprouts have been included in the diet—and medicine—of dozens of cultures from East to West. The use of sprouts is even older than the Bible. In this chapter we will discuss some of the ways sprouts were and are used by traditional peoples, and trace their recent popularity in America and the Western World.

Ancient manuscripts show us that by about 3000 B.C., the Chinese were eating bean sprouts on a regular basis. The Emperor of China at that time also recorded certain therapeutic uses of sprouts in a book about medicinal herbs. He indicated that sprouted beans could help cure such diverse problems as bloating, loss of nerve sensation, muscular cramps, digestive disorders, and weakness of the lungs.

In the late sixteenth century, Li Shih Chen's *Pen Ts'ao Kang Mu*, an exhaustive work on Chinese pharmaceuticals and herbs which took over twenty-six years to complete, also discussed the medicinal value of sprouts. Chen suggested them for use in reducing inflammation, obtaining a laxative effect, remedying dropsy and rheumatism, and building and toning the body.

The Chinese and other Far Eastern peoples still use mung, ad-zuki, soy, wheat, and barley for sprouting as part of their daily diet.

In the book *Healthy Hunzas*, John Tobe reports that the long-lived natives of this mountainous Asian region use sprouts for survival during the long, cold winters. In the spring, before crops have matured and after much of their stored food has been eaten, the Hunzas rely on sprouts as a source of vitamins, enzymes, and energy.

In the West, during the eighteenth century, British sailor Captain James Cook first tested the antiscorbutic (anti-scurvy) properties of sprouts. Scurvy, caused by a lack of ascorbic acid (vitamin C), is first apparent as lowered resistance to infection and a tendency to bleed easily. In severe cases it leads to weakness, weight loss, painfully swollen joints, bleeding gums, loosened teeth, and bleeding under the skin. Cook and his crew used a specially formulated malt made by cooking sprouted beans at a very low heat for long periods. Captain Cook sailed the seas for over three years without losing a single man to the wasting disease.

Until Cook's voyage, most ships on extended journeys lost an average of half their crews to scurvy. The British Navy tried a variety of measures to combat the problem, including growing gardens on the decks of ships, and brewing unpasteurized beers and ales—the latter leading to many a navigational error! And after it was discovered that citrus fruits such as lemons also prevented scurvy, Captain Cook's sprout concoction was no longer used.

The menace of scurvy remained several centuries later. The plight of British and Indian troops in Mesopotamia during World War I attracted the attention of researchers who found a simple but effective solution. Knowing that vegetables, greens, and legumes (beans and peas), once dried, could not prevent scurvy, they experimented with fresh pea and bean sprouts. Even though transporting fresh vegetables or lemons to the front was next to impossible, sprouting was quite feasible.

A British doctor named John Wiltshire put both lemons and sprouted beans to the test to see which could cure scurvy faster, with less expense and bother. His experiment consisted of treating sixty patients suffering from scurvy in a Serbian hospital. One group was fed four ounces of fresh lemon juice daily, and the other was given four ounces of sprouted haricot beans. The sprouted beans and lemon juice contained equal amounts of vitamin C. After a month, the sprout-fed patients showed a greater rate of improvement than those fed the lemon juice. In addition, treatment with sprouts was found to be less expensive to administer. When the experiment ended, with all sixty patients discharged, the physician recommended the use of sprouted beans as the easiest and cheapest method to prevent scurvy in the field.

In India, during 1938, severe crop failures and food shortages were responsible for thousands of deaths due to scurvy and famine. It wasn't until January 1940 that a plan that aimed to solve the problem was announced. Each of the over 200,000 people in the program was given an ounce of dried sprouted grain or chick peas twice a week. After four months of sprout rationing there were no reported cases of scurvy, and by the end of April the plan was deemed no longer necessary. However, by the end of September 1940—during the five months that followed the program—there were over a thousand more deaths due to scurvy than there had been the year before. In January 1941 the sprouting program was reintroduced, this time to 140,000 people. Once again, scurvy cases dropped to nil after four months.

In addition to providing enough vitamin C to prevent scurvy, sprouts can supply adequate amounts of protein to maintain health. During World War II, Dr. Clive McCay of Cornell University's school of nutrition was one of the researchers who sought alternative protein sources for Americans. It was feared that the war might bring shortages of meat, poultry, dairy foods, and other staple proteins, as it had in Europe. The alternative Dr. McCay came up with was sprouted seeds, beans, and grains, especially the protein-rich soybean. A campaign was then launched by the U.S. government to teach Americans how to grow and use sprouted beans and seeds. Books and cookbooks all about sprouting were published and distributed throughout the United States by the Government Printing Office. But the expected protein shortages never came, and by 1945 sprouts were forgotten by almost everyone.

Even though sprouts didn't catch on during the war, they have recently gained increased popularity. According to a study by O. B. Hesterman and L. R. Teuber, both at the University of California at Davis, people in the United States are eating more sprouts than ever before. In California, their report states, there was a seventeen-fold increase in the use of alfalfa sprouts between 1970 and 1979. More than 10 million pounds of alfalfa sprouts are produced by California growers each year. And this figure doesn't account for the many people who grow their own sprouts.

Today you can find sprouts in almost any supermarket. Sprouts have been instrumental in popularizing the spread of salad bars. Lately, they have even been showing up on the sandwiches of the major fast food chains. New sprout-growing businesses are popping up all over, some of them producing more than 15,000 pounds of sprouts per day, and doing more than $1½ million of business a year. A number of types of manual and automatic home sprout growers are on the market, and there is even a newsletter called *The Sproutletter*, which is almost entirely devoted to educating readers about sprouting.

Since the 1950s, when I began promoting the use of sprouts in America and abroad, many new organizations have formed to help spread the message of sprouting. At the Ann Wigmore Foundation, we receive dozens of letters every week asking about sprouts and the Living Food Lifestyle.

Touted for many years as a "future food" by conservative nutritionists, it's clear that sprouts have arrived, and are here to stay. The reason is simple; few foods today require as little time, energy, and expense to produce yet yield so much nutrition. When used in abundance, sprouts have the power to keep your body young by giving your cells high-quality nourishment and helping to cleanse them of toxic wastes.

In Chapter 2 we will begin our discussion of why sprouts are so good for us, focusing first of all on their nutritional values.

2

From Seed to Nutritious Food

The germinating seed represents a protein manufacturing machine which is turning out protein . . . along with the necessary vitamins and minerals for its assimilation and utilization.

Dr. Jeffrey Bland,
Biochemist, University of Puget Sound

At the foundation of the living foods concept is the seed. Filled with nutrients needed by the growing plant, and suffused with vital enzymes, seeds are the very core of life. All the energy and life of a plant goes toward making seeds. Each seed holds vitamins, minerals, proteins, fats, and carbohydrates (starches) in reserve, awaiting the suitable environment to begin growing. When air, water, and a suitable temperature are provided, a miracle begins. When the seed germinates (begins to sprout) an incredible flow of energy is released. Natural chemical changes occur. Enzymes are produced to convert the concentrated nutrients into those needed by the growing plant.

As the sprouting process continues, carbohydrates are transformed by the action of enzymes into simple sugars. Complex proteins are converted into more simple amino acids and fats are changed into fatty acids, which are easily digested soluble compounds. Vitamin C, along with some other vitamins found only in trace amounts in the seed, is produced in larger amounts during sprouting. In addition, sprouts absorb minerals and vital trace elements from the water used to grow and rinse them. Moreover, the minerals in sprouts are chelated; that is, in their natural state, they are chemically bound to amino acids, so that they are easily assimilated by the human body.

ENZYMES AND VITAL FOOD FACTORS IN SPROUTS

Enzymes are greatly activated in the sprouting process. Just minutes after raw unsprouted seeds are placed in water to soak, enzymes begin making the young sprouts into easy-to-digest food for humans. In sprouts, as in other uncooked foods, all the nutrients work together in natural harmony and balance for optimal use by the human body. Cooking destroys this balance, breaking down the molecular arrangement of nutrients. Enzymes are destroyed by temperatures over 105° F, as are a large percentage of the vitamins in foods. Minerals in cooked food are no longer chelated, and are therefore more difficult for the body to use. Protein is also damaged by cooking, as the amino acid ratios become unbalanced. Cooked protein foods (especially animal foods such as red meat and eggs) tend to putrefy and decay, producing toxic wastes that must be removed from the body by the kidneys. Proteins from sprouts and other uncooked foods produce fewer toxic substances during digestion.

Beyond enzymes, which are a valuable aid to digestion, sprouts contain what I call *vital food factors*—the energy currents that flow through all living bodies and differentiate them from dead bodies. While little hard data has been collected on just how and why the vital food factors found primarily in sprouts and other living foods affect human health, my own experience and observation of thousands of other people points to an amazing ability of sprouts to regenerate body cells and tissues. The vital food factors in sprouts and other living foods are released from plant cells during the process of chewing and digestion, and become usable for the regeneration of the human body.

Sprouts are biogenic—they are alive. And I am convinced that a carload of cooked food cannot do for the healing and regeneration of the human body what a single sprouted seed will do. Imagine a farmer cooking seeds before sowing them! For that matter—can you picture in your mind any food in your present diet that, when planted, will sprout and grow up to create a new life? Cooked grains, beans, or vegetables won't. Neither will animal foods such as meat, eggs, and cheese. Only uncooked germinated seeds, grains, nuts, and beans can give us their living energy.

AMINO ACIDS (PROTEINS) IN SPROUTS

Plant proteins are the highest-quality proteins available, and sprouts are loaded with them. Plant proteins are easy for the body to use, are low in fat, and contain no saturated fats or cholesterol. In contrast, the proteins in animal foods are generally associated with large quantities of potentially harmful fats, and are more difficult for the body to assimilate. Animal foods, especially when they have been cooked, tend to produce toxic waste products when they are broken down during the course of normal digestion.

Among the sprouts, lentils are the richest single source of high-quality protein. Seven cups of sprouted lentils contain approximately 58 grams of protein—more than enough to meet the U.S. RDA (Recommended Daily Allowance) for an adult male!

Proteins are constructed of building blocks called amino acids. There are eight essential amino acids: isoleucine, leucine, lysine, methionine, phenylalanine, threonine, tryptophane, and valine—which the body must synthesize from the proteins we eat. When these eight are not provided in the diet, the body is unable to regenerate its cells properly and deficiency symptoms arise. The fourteen other amino acids are actually just as essential, but can be formed by the body internally.

Amino acids act on the blood and body cells in the process of self-renewal that rejuvenates us and prolongs life. They are important to so many body functions and systems it would be impossible to list them all here. We can summarize their effect by stating that they are essential to proper digestion and assimilation of foods, cell renewal, immunity from disease and illness, rapid healing of cuts and wounds, and proper liver function.

A deficiency of only one amino acid can result in allergies, low energy levels, poor digestion, lowered resistance, and premature aging. The replacement of the missing amino acid can as easily result in a complete reversal of these symptoms.

Amino acids are found in abundant variety in all living foods. Sprouted seeds, beans, grains, and nuts provide complete proteins—that is, they will give you all eight essential amino acids. It is best, however, to eat a variety of sprouts, as each kind has a different proportion of amino acids.

In essence, the amino acids supplied by sprouts can make the difference between fair health and below-average energy levels —and overall well-being and vitality.

VITAMINS IN SPROUTS

The question of whether we need nutritional supplements, including vitamins, is hotly debated—needlessly. Vitamins are essential nutrients that regulate chemical reactions in the body. They help to make the energy present in food available to our cells. And all of the vitamins necessary for health are supplied abundantly when plenty of sprouts and living foods are eaten.

The majority of supplemental vitamins are synthesized from coal tar and other petroleum derivatives. And while they may appear to be chemically identical to natural vitamins, they may have only a fraction of the biological activity, making them poor substitutes for their natural counterparts. Synthetics may also have additional, harmful effects. Vitamin manufacturers warn us that large doses of supplemental vitamins A, B complex, C, D, and E can hurt us.

The vitamins found in fresh sprouts and other living foods are completely safe and are capable of sustaining us in good health as long as enough of the right kinds of foods are eaten. Humans have gotten vitamins this way for millions of years. I recommend the use of several cups of sprouts a day in salads, blended soups, and other dishes.

Right up until the moment you eat a fresh raw sprout, it is growing and increasing in nutritional value. The nutrients remain intact until you begin chewing. Whereas other living foods, such as fresh vegetables, contain ample supplies of vitamins, their nutrient values begin to steadily decline as soon as they are cut. The vitamin C contained in a crushed raw radish, for example, decreases by half in about five minutes, and by up to seventy percent in twenty minutes. In cooking, much of the vitamin (and mineral) content of fresh foods is lost—thrown out with the cooking water, or oxidized (see page 20) by exposure to air and heat.

Amazingly, raw, unsprouted lentil seeds have too low a vitamin C level to measure, but after sprouting their vitamin C level increases enough to make them one of the better sources of it. Vitamin C is important to the health of the skin, teeth, and gums. It also aids in growth and development, and protects other vitamins from oxidation. Nutritionally, fresh lentil, cabbage, mung, and adzuki bean sprouts are good sources of vitamin C. Sprouted chick peas and cow peas also contain this vitamin.

Alfalfa sprouts are not only a good source of vitamin C, but a provider of vitamin A as well. In fact, they have more vitamin A than is found in comparable amounts of tomatoes, lettuce, green peppers, and most fruits. The sprouts are rich in vitamin A, containing up to four times more than raw, unsprouted seeds. Sprouted cabbage, clover, peas, and mustard are also excellent sources of vitamin A. The vitamin A in sprouts is supplied to us in the form of carotene, which is converted into vitamin A in the intestine as needed. Carotene is non-toxic in large quantities, whereas synthetic vitamin A or that found in fish oils, liver, and other animal foods, accumulates in the liver and can become toxic. Vitamin A is essential for normal growth and development, for good eyesight, and in reproduction.

The B vitamins thiamine (B_1), riboflavin (B_2), and niacin are abundant in sprouted almond, alfalfa, wheat, rye, sunflower, and sesame. Sunflower and sesame sprouts are richer in these important B vitamins than are raw, unsprouted seeds (which by themselves are considered to be a good source of B vitamins). The vitamin B complex helps the body digest carbohydrates and use the energy in them, and also promotes resistance to infection. Moreover, the B complex, sometimes called the "stress vitamins," aids the normal functioning of the nervous system, thus bolstering it against stress of all kinds.

Wheat is one of the best sources of vitamin E, which functions as an antioxidant, preventing valuable nutrients from being destroyed or wasted. In addition, this vitamin is a protector of the heart and a fertility tonic. Sprouting wheat increases its vitamin E content by three times over that of the raw, unsprouted seed. In addition, the type of vitamin E found in sprouted seeds, grains, and nuts—such as oats, rye, alfalfa, sesame, sunflower, and almonds—is at least ten times more easily assimilated by the body than synthetic E. I will have more to say about vitamin E and sprouts in the next chapter.

Vitamin K is found in abundance in alfalfa sprouts. This little-known vitamin is especially important during pregnancy, as it is responsible for blood clotting, and aids in the prevention of hemorrhages and miscarriages. Vitamin U, another lesser-known vitamin, is found in abundance in cabbage sprouts. It is currently being investigated for its potential to prevent stomach and intestinal ulcers.

MINERALS AND TRACE ELEMENTS IN SPROUTS

Dietary minerals are our lifeblood. They serve as the foundation for the body's overall metabolism—the vital chemical and physical processes that keep the body functioning smoothly. Minerals figure in the formation and function of all body enzymes, and also keep the proper alkaline electrical charge in all the body cells, guarding them against acidic degeneration and invasion from harmful microbes that live on acidic substances in the body.

Over two billion years ago, minerals in the ancient ocean mixed with amino acids and enzymes and made life forms. The complex mineral salts found in plants and animals are responsible for the transmission of electrical current through the living organism. These mineral salts are organic minerals, as opposed to the inorganic minerals found in stone, a rusty nail, or in many mineral supplements.

While studies have indicated that some inorganic minerals can be used by the body to serve a specified function, you need to take ten to twenty times more concentrated doses than those found in foods to get the desired effect. Unfortunately, the added quantities of minerals also create a risk of overload. The Bantu people of Africa, for example, have a high incidence of poisoning due to their exclusive use of iron pots and pans for cooking. The excess iron is stored in the liver and causes a toxic reaction that can result in death. Excesses of minerals other than iron can also create a chaotic condition in the body, by upsetting the delicate balance among minerals.

To meet your body's needs for minerals such as calcium, potassium, iron, phosphorus, and magnesium, sanely and safely, I recommend you get them from sprouts and other living foods in the form of organic mineral salts. This is the way humans have been fulfilling mineral needs for millennia.

Sprouts are an especially good source of easy-to-use minerals. Research by Dr. Jeffrey Bland at the University of Puget Sound has shown that sprouts absorb minerals and trace elements (minerals needed in small amounts, such as iodine, zinc, or selenium) from the water used to rinse them while they are growing. In addition, minerals and trace elements found in the raw, unsprouted seeds become more digestible through the sprouting process.

Sesame sprouts are an exceptionally good source of calcium, having about as much of this vital mineral as cow's milk, and more than almost any other plant food. Almond, sunflower, alfalfa, and chick pea sprouts are also excellent sources of calcium in organic form. Ninety-nine percent of the calcium we eat is deposited in our bones and teeth, keeping them healthy and strong.

Potassium is sometimes called the "youth mineral" because it helps the body to maintain smooth and tight skin and balanced body weight. It also helps to maintain the proper alkalinity of the blood. Almond, sesame, sunflower, mung, and cow pea sprouts supply more potassium than many fruits and garden vegetables.

Alfalfa, fenugreek, lentil, adzuki, and mung sprouts are good sources of the iron needed for red blood cell formation and the transport of oxygen from the lungs to the cells. Sprouted seeds are also rich in iron. Even though some of our iron is recycled internally, we need to get additional iron in organic form from our food. This is especially true for women, who may develop iron deficiencies due to menstrual blood loss.

In general, sprouts are excellent sources of trace elements such as iodine, zinc, selenium, chromium, cobalt, and silicon. Alfalfa sprouts and sprouted pumpkin seeds are especially potent sources of zinc, which is essential for the synthesis of protein, for many liver functions, and in the healing of cuts and wounds. Selenium, which is now being tested for anti-cancer properties, is also supplied by many sprouts, especially alfalfa.

CHLOROPHYLL IN SPROUTS

One of the most important nutrient compounds contained in sprouts, chlorophyll, has been thoroughly researched for its nutritional and healing properties. By itself, chlorophyll, a protein compound found in green plants, including sprouts with green leaves (such as alfalfa, cabbage, clover, sunflower, and radish), doesn't appear to be anything special. But there are two vital aspects of chlorophyll that shouldn't be overlooked.

First is its creation in the plant as a result of a conversion of the sun's energy—which makes it a sort of living battery; and second is its remarkable similarity to a vital component of human blood—hemoglobin. Circulating in the bloodstream, hemoglobin molecules carry oxygen to the cells throughout the body.

Unlike humans and animals, who get energy from food, plants get their energy directly from the sun. Plants create and store carbohydrate energy as a result of the sun's action upon their leaves, in the process known as photosynthesis. In fresh green sprouts, this energy is readily available to the human body for healing and regeneration of the cells.

Moreover, the chemical elements contained in chlorophyll are effective in building up the red blood cell content of the bloodstream. Exactly how and why this can occur is still largely unknown, but many theories have been offered. The chlorophyll molecule is quite similar to hemoglobin. The main difference is that chlorophyll has a magnesium ion as a nucleus, whereas hemoglobin is structured around iron.

Dr. Yoshihide Hagiwara, a Japanese scientist who researches the healing power of green plants and grasses, feels that scientists will soon discover that chlorophyll is converted into blood inside us. He reasons that since chlorophyll is soluble in fat particles, and since fat particles are absorbed directly into the blood via the lymphatic system, that chlorophyll can also be absorbed in this way. It is his opinion that once the chlorophyll molecule is absorbed, its magnesium ion is replaced with iron, making new hemoglobin.

Enzymes and vital food factors, proteins, vitamins, minerals, and chlorophyll—the nutritional benefits of including fresh sprouts in the diet are numerous. We will discuss some of the health benefits in the next chapter.

3

Sprouting and Health

The more we exploit nature, the more our options are reduced,
until we only have one: to fight for survival.

Morris Udall

Science is only beginning to penetrate the mysteries of life energies in living things, but scientists will soon recognize what I've been witnessing for over two dozen years at the health center I've founded and directed. Regeneration and rejuvenation of the human body *is* possible, when it is given a rest from destructive habits and supplied with foods rich in life energy. Moreover, serious degenerative conditions may be controlled, and in some cases even reversed, when positive changes in diet and lifestyle are made.

The life energy in fresh sprouts stimulates the body's inherent self-cleansing and self-healing abilities. Particularly when the body is freed from the debilitating effects of cooked, heavy foods, the natural processes that work in the healing of a cut or the lowering of a fever can also be put to work healing and revitalizing the internal workings of the body. This was demonstrated in an experiment performed by M. L. Armstrong et al., and reported in the journal *Circulation Research* in 1970. Advanced cholesterol buildup in the arteries of Rhesus monkeys was caused by a high-cholesterol, high-fat experimental diet, and *reversed* with a low-fat, low-cholesterol diet. We are now beginning to see the same results in studies of humans as well. And if serious illnesses like heart disease can be reversed and controlled, then why can't other cripplers like cancer also be controlled and even reversed? After years of experience in working with ill persons, I have come to believe that serious degenerative conditions can be controlled and in some cases reversed, but central to my conviction is that the individual must make positive changes in his or her attitude and lifestyle. Specifically, a diet rich in foods abundantly supplied with life energy, and a happy, confident, and relaxed outlook.

CAN SPROUTS HELP CONTROL CANCER?

Thelma Arthur, M.D., of the Arthur Testing Labs in Chula Vista, California, studied nearly two hundred of my guests before and after they followed the Living Food Lifestyle for at least two weeks. She was especially interested in the effect of this diet as she believes it may hold an answer to cancer control. She was curious as to why components of the diet—sprouts, wheatgrass, fresh juices, and a variety of raw foods—are being used by several wholistic health centers, and why individuals such as Eydie Mae Hunsburger survived cancer illnesses while eating this way.

Dr. Arthur's conclusions showed significant increases in the body's immune response—its ability to fight off illness—in nearly every case. The toxicity level of the blood, which is usually high in illnesses such as cancer, was reduced in nearly every case. This is not to say that sprouts by themselves can reverse or even control cancer and other serious illness. It may, however, point to the ability of sprouts, living foods, and wheatgrass to strengthen the immune system, which should be the aim of any sane approach to the problem of cancer. For even though a given therapy may destroy cancer cells, if it weakens the immune system greatly at the same time, a simple infection or a common cold can turn into a deadly enemy.

In 1978, at the University of Texas Cancer Center, Dr. Charles Shaw and Dr. Chiu-Nan Lai tested a variety of vegetable foods for potential anti-cancer elements. Among the foods tested on mice inoculated with carcinogens (cancer-causing substances) were lentil, mung, and wheat sprouts, and carrots and parsley. Whereas the carrots and parsley did show an inhibitory effect on carcinogens, they weren't nearly as potent as the sprouts were in terms of anti-cancer activity!

Their research results were of particular interest to medical and cancer researchers for two reasons: the inhibited activity of carcinogens was quite strong, even when reasonably small dosages of a sprout extract were used, and the extract was not toxic even in high dosage. (Most known inhibitors of carcinogens are toxic at even moderately high levels of concentration.) While this experiment in no way represents conclusive proof that sprouts can cure cancer in humans, the outlook for further research into the use of sprouts as anti-cancer foods is promising indeed. It is also worth noting that the beneficial effects sprouts have on the immune system may be enhanced by other elements of the Living Food program, in particular, by the consumption of easily digestible blended foods.

SPROUTS: THE IDEAL COMPANION FOR DIETERS

The problem of overweight, and its solution, has become needlessly complicated. Some experts tell us that diets don't work; others say they do. I am absolutely sure that the right diet does work. In the final analysis, permanent weight loss can only be achieved by eating the right kinds of foods, and when necessary by eating less food. Regular exercise is also important, but in my opinion, diet is the main component of successful weight loss.

In terms of day-to-day living, the energy required to carry excess weight around and to feed pockets of fat is great. Yet that same energy is needed in order to be disciplined about eating and exercising right. When an abundance of sprouts (along with other live foods) is included in the diet, the overweight person gets a much-needed rest.

Sprouts, particularly alfalfa, supply the body with a large quantity of low-calorie liquid nourishment that is easily digested and used as fuel. The body's internal self-cleansing abilities are stimulated by sprouts and sprout juices, and overall metabolism is speeded up because it isn't weighed down by lots of hard-to-digest food. In addition, the liquids help to flush toxins out of the body.

These benefits of my weight loss program are the complete opposite of the effects of some weight loss plans. In particular, high-protein diets tie up the body's energy reserves in order to convert large quantities of building foods (proteins) into energy foods (carbohydrates). The high-protein dieter is usually exhausted after a few weeks.

With the Living Food Lifestyle, there is an average weight loss of four to fifteen pounds per week, while the individual eats three filling meals per day. Easy-to-digest, nutritious, and cleansing sprouts, greens, and other living foods are the key. For example, various sprouts may be juiced with fruits and vegetables to make delightful "green drinks."

The pungent, cleansing sprouts radish, fenugreek, cabbage, alfalfa, and clover are especially good for weight loss. Nevertheless, it is important to include a variety of foods in your diet when you are trying to lose weight. Sprouted grains such as wheat are a sensible choice because they are rich in energy and have cleansing properties too. Buckwheat and sunflower greens (see Chapter 7) are also good choices, as they are high in liquid content and easy to digest.

SPROUTS AND YOUR SEX LIFE

What do sprouts have to do with your sex life? Perhaps little if your sex life is already satisfying. On the other hand, they could do a lot to improve unsatisfactory relationships—restoring sexual desire and performance to their normal healthy state.

It is common sense that when you are more healthy physically, *all* parts of you are more healthy. When you and your mate look and feel better, sexual attraction is enhanced. While I have received much feedback from guests on positive changes in their sexual lives once they've adopted the Living Food Lifestyle, much of the scientific evidence for sprouts affecting sexual functioning comes from, of all places, the barnyard.

In numerous studies of cattle, the addition of sprouts to the diet was found to increase the production of milk in cows and to restore fertility to cows that were sterile. This is not surprising because wheat sprouts, for example, supply more and better-quality vitamin E than does wheat germ—a noted source of the fertility vitamin.

Although wheat is one of the highest sources of natural vitamin E, its content of E triples when it is sprouted. Other sprouted grains, notably oats and rye, are also excellent sources of vitamin E, as are all sprouted seeds and nuts.

Years ago, experiments performed by the Agricultural Experiment Station in Beltsville, Maryland, demonstrated the ability of sprouted grains to restore fertility to cows that lost or outgrew their ability to reproduce. In one study involving cows that had never reproduced, even though breeding had been attempted, each animal was fed five pounds of sprouted oats along with its regular food each day. The results were amazing. After just sixty days all the cows were made pregnant.

The point of these studies is that sexual functions can be rejuvenated and restored to their normal healthy state when the diet includes an abundance of sprouts.

SLOWING THE AGING CLOCK
WITH SPROUTS

That sprouts can slow down or even reverse aging may seem farfetched. But recent publications about longevity and nutrition indicate that they can, in more ways than one. A number of nutrients have been cited as potential anti-aging factors by Durk Pearson and Sandy Shaw, Dr. Benjamin Frank, Dr. Edward Howell, and others.

Some anti-aging nutrients that have received attention include antioxidants and a broad range of exogenous enzymes (enzymes that come from a source outside the body). While it is true that many factors may affect aging, a balanced living foods diet, with plenty of fresh sprouts, offers you a completely safe source of potential anti-aging nutrients. Sprouts contain the natural antioxidant vitamins, A, C, and E, along with exogenous enzymes.

Antioxidants in Sprouts

Oxidation is a type of chemical reaction that can have either a damaging or a beneficial effect in terms of nutrition. When substances are oxidized outside the human body, they are damaged or destroyed. When foods are broken down *inside* the body during the course of normal digestion, oxidation also takes place—the vital difference is that the food energy is made available for our use. Yet another aspect of oxidation relates to the formation of "free radicals."

Lately there has been much talk among health advocates of "free radicals" and their damaging effects on human health. Free radicals are molecular fragments with a bunch of wild electrons that can surround your cells internally and age every part of your body in the process. They are very unstable and tend to disrupt the normal activity of anything they get close to. Unfortunately, free radicals are created by the processed oils and cooked fats in the modern diet.

Antioxidants such as vitamins A, C, and E prevent the oxidation of fats in the blood, thus inhibiting the formation of free radicals in the body. Vitamin C not only prevents free radicals from being formed, but also keeps vitamins A and E from being destroyed. Although vitamin A is not found in any plant food, its precursor, carotene, is. Carotene prevents the oils in plants from becoming free radicals while the plants are still alive.

Sprouts and living foods are excellent sources of antioxidants. In addition, limiting or avoiding altogether the use of processed oils and cooked fats will help prevent the formation of free radicals, thus preventing premature aging of the body.

Food Enzymes Abound in Sprouts

Enzymes, along with water, are the substances that distinguish sprouts from raw, unsprouted seeds. It is the activity of enzymes that converts starches into sugars, proteins into amino acids, and fats into fatty acids inside the sprout. Enzymes also function within the human digestive system to break down food so that its nutrients may be easily used by the body. When exogenous enzymes are not present in foods—as is the case with cooked and processed foods—the body must supply the missing enzymes. In other words, it is forced to produce more protein-splitting enzymes (proteases), more starch-splitting enzymes (amylases), and more fat-splitting enzymes (lipases) than it would if the foods themselves contained these enzymes.

According to the pioneering enzymologist Edward Howell, M.D., the author of *Enzyme Nutrition*, youthfulness depends upon the quantity and strength of enzymes present in the body. The more endogenous (internal) enzymes the digestive system requires to break down food, he explains, the lower the inner reserves of metabolic enzymes. This is significant because metabolic enzymes play a crucial role in countless body processes. In advanced age, reserves of metabolic enzymes are at their lowest level, and the strength of digestive enzymes is diminished as well. Dr. Howell concludes that the faster we use up our supply of endogenous enzymes—the more cooked, enzymeless food we consume—the quicker we age. The aging process accelerates as the body is compelled to draw upon its already-depleted reserves of metabolic enzymes. At this writing, Dr. Howell is eighty-seven years old and, as he has for many years, tries to eat as much of his food as possible raw.

When sprouts are eaten raw, they are a good source of important food enzymes that aid in the digestion of starch, protein, and fat. Cellulase, a food enzyme that works on cellulose, is also present in sprouts. The more concentrated a sprout is in a given substance, the more of the particular enzyme required to help break it down will be present. So lentils, which are relatively high in protein, are more rich in protease than, for example, chick peas, which contain more starch, and therefore more amylase.

The food enzymes in sprouts not only work to digest themselves, but help the body to digest other foods as well. Humans (and their domesticated animals) are the only creatures on earth who eat their food without its natural enzymes (i.e., cooked). Dr. Howell believes that this is one reason why people suffer from cancer and other degenerative conditions that animals in the wild are free from, and my years of experience working in the health care field lead me to the same conclusion.

In fact, food enzymes are the key to the effectiveness of the Living Food Lifestyle, for they carry the vital life energy from sprouts and other live foods into the body. The abundance of food enzymes in these biogenic and bioactive foods is what separates them from all other foods. Fresh raw sprouts are alive and at their peak of nutritional value just before they are eaten. Once they have been consumed, they help digest themselves, thereby giving the body a much-needed rest, and enabling it to begin regenerating and repairing itself.

Enzyme-rich foods such as sprouts, fresh vegetables, fruits, and their juices, are the most important factors in slowing the aging clock. Meats and other heavy, cooked foods, especially those that are also fatty or sugary, are deficient in food enzymes. These foods slow the rate of body metabolism and weaken the immune system. As we have seen, live foods help the body to conserve its vital enzymes, stimulating metabolism and the cleansing/regenerative process. In this way, as well as by inhibiting potential carcinogens, live foods, particularly sprouts, have the capacity to strengthen the immune system and help us to lead long and healthy lives.

4

The Economics of Sprouting

All work is as seed sown; it grows and spreads, and sows itself anew.

Thomas Carlyle

While it is difficult to place a value on a food as healthful as sprouts, it's easy to price them. Pound for pound sprouts are perhaps the most nutritious food there is per dollar value. Buckwheat and sunflower greens are economical, too. This is due in part to the fact that sprouts and indoor greens increase in size, weight, and nutritional value as they grow. In addition, there is an abundance of seeds all over the world available for sprouting.

COST OF SPROUTS PER POUND

The costs, weights, and yields of thirty different kinds of seeds have been carefully assessed by editor Jeff Breakey in *The Sproutletter*, a newsletter devoted to sprouting. Of all these familiar—and some not-so-common—seeds, wheat, buckwheat, and sunflower grown on soil (see Chapter 7) were the least expensive per food value dollar. On the average, it costs a little over 13 cents per pound to grow these greens at home.

The popular sprout alfalfa costs only 33 cents a pound, while its weight from seed to sprout increases over 600 percent and its volume increases by 2900 percent. In Breakey's study, one pound of alfalfa seeds produced nearly seven pounds of alfalfa sprouts.

Mung or Chinese bean sprouts cost 28 cents per pound and increase in volume more than ten times. You can grow a variety of sprouts that will provide you with the Recommended Daily Allowance of protein, vitamins, and minerals, and, as Breakey points out, you can grow them for less than one dollar per day (see the list that follows). To get the same amount of nutrients from meat, even if it were possible, would cost a small fortune—and the same holds true for bee pollen, algae, and other so-called super health foods.

Serving Size (cups)	Variety	Seed Price (cents per serving)
½	almond sprouts	26
½	sesame sprouts	8
1½	wheat sprouts	6
1	rye sprouts	3.5
1	sunflower sprouts	14.5
3	alfalfa sprouts	9
1½	lentil sprouts	6.5
2	mung sprouts	8.5
3	buckwheat sprouts	2.5
3	sunflower greens	5
3	wheatgrass (juiced)	2.5
20		92.0

From *The Sproutletter*, Ashland, Oregon, Issue No. 14, Jan.–Feb., 1983. Reprinted by permission.

Of course, I'm not recommending that you attempt to live entirely on sprouts. The addition of fermented seed and nut cheeses, fresh and dried fruits, vegetables such as avocados, and sprouted breads are important sources of calories that can be lacking in a diet based on sprouts. But clearly the use of sprouts rests on a firm economic basis, not only for consumption in this country, but also in famine-stricken parts of the world, where sprouted seeds and grains could be used to alleviate nutritional deficiencies.

HEALING CAMPS IN INDIA

In the past fifteen years I made several trips to the large cities of India to set up healing camps with doctors and government administrators there. Hundreds of people with all sorts of problems—from heart disease and cancer to leprosy and malnutrition—were admitted to these camps. The patients stayed in the camp and ate sprouts, wheatgrass, and other living foods until they recovered. The recovery of starving children who were placed on a diet combining sprouts and fruits was truly amazing. In less than thirty days, their sores and scars disappeared, and abdominal swelling was in every case reduced to normal. Above all, these children became able to run and play, instead of having to be carried around by their mothers because they were unable to walk on their own.

Of course, in many parts of the world, the problem isn't so much what people eat (they are so poor they cannot afford meat, milk, and the various junk foods that are so detrimental to the health of people in this country), but how little they eat. Yet, when some of the poorest people in India were given a choice of foods, they most often chose meat and milk, perhaps a result of having been misled into believing that these are the most nutritious foods. Nevertheless, they soon learned that sprouts could easily be grown at home as an inexpensive way to supplement their diet (primarily local fruits, vegetables, grains, and beans). Even now research is continuing to determine which sprouts are best for use in India, and to develop the best ways to educate people about growing and preparing sprouts for themselves at home.

FRESH SPROUTS VERSUS DRIED

For some time there has been talk of using flours made from dried sprouted grains, beans, and seeds as a protein supplement that could be added to bread or made into meat analogues. Whereas a fresh sprouted wheatberry contains about 3 or 4 percent protein, dried wheatgrass contains up to 45 percent protein. Yet, drying wheatberries and other sprouts de-

stroys some of their valuable enzymes and drives their life
energy from them—making them little better, healthwise, than
ordinary flour.

We would be much better off using fresh sprouts instead of
dried sprout flours. There are millions of pounds of surplus
grains and other seeds that could be sprouted and distributed
where there are shortages of food, and where few fresh vegetables and fruits are available. My experience with the healing
camps in India has convinced me of the benefits that these
sprouts can provide, and I hope that they will soon be used to
help malnourished people everywhere.

Seeds should also be put to use for sprouting in the affluent
West, where under the guise of plenty we too are suffering—
from junk foods, and the lack of vital life energy in them. The
use of sprouts and living foods can make a vast difference in
our health. While many of us are unaware of it, we may suffer
from symptoms of malnutrition. Research by the U.S. Depart-
ment of Agriculture, published as the *Nationwide Food Comparison Survey 1977–78*, showed that Americans may not be getting
enough calcium, iron, vitamin A, and B-complex vitamins in
their diet. Though we drink more milk, and eat more cheese
and red meat (all supposed to be good sources of calcium or
iron), than any other nation, we still aren't getting enough of
these nutrients. A daily glass of orange juice and a serving of
overcooked canned or frozen vegetables do not supply enough
vitamins A and C. Modern food processing and refining
methods strip the valuable germ and bran from our breads,
noodles, breakfast cereals, and other grain products, depleting
their stores of B-complex vitamins, and making inefficient and
costly (and risky, from a health point of view) supplementation
of grain products necessary.

Although sprout growers on the west coast of the United
States are reporting huge increases in the production and sale
of alfalfa and mung sprouts over the past five years, I hope that
many more people will begin growing sprouts—at home. Far-
reaching economic benefits await us when we begin to reduce
our dependence upon costly and unhealthful animal proteins,
because at present animal husbandry is squandering a huge
percentage of the world's energy and potential food resources.

In sum, sprouts provide people everywhere with the protein and supplemental nutrients necessary to facilitate a smooth transition from a diet based on animal foods to a more healthful—and more economical—vegetable-based one.

5

Shopper's Guide to Sprouting Seeds

Fruits ripen, not to make food for us, but to protect the seeds inside. But we pay no attention to Nature's purpose, and enjoy the delicate flavors and delicious flesh of apples, pears, peaches, tomatoes, melons, and all, and throw aside carelessly the seeds that the plant went to so much trouble to build, and in which it stored the life-giving germ and a reserve of starch to help it start in life again as a baby plant.

Luther Burbank

When it comes to sprouting, not all seeds are created equal. As a result of nearly thirty years of sprouting seeds (including nuts and beans), I have learned which ones sprout most easily and are most flavorful as sprouts. This chapter will describe my favorite sprouts, focusing on their nutritional highlights and uses. Guidelines for choosing and buying seeds are also provided, because the quality of the seeds you use to sprout is as important as the method you use to sprout them. Growing methods are the subject of the next chapter.

Adzuki beans are small red beans (similar in size to mung beans) that have been cultivated for centuries in China, Japan, Korea, and other Far Eastern countries. They are also grown in the United States, and are available at most natural foods stores and Oriental markets here.

Sprouted adzuki beans contain amino acids (protein), vitamin C, and iron, among other nutrients. Their flavor resembles that of mung bean sprouts. Use sprouted adzuki beans in salads, Chinese-style marinated vegetables, green drinks, sprout loaves, and sandwiches. Adzuki sprouts are versatile due to their mild flavor and crunchy texture.

Alfalfa seeds are small, about the size of a pinhead, and tan in color. Often considered to be a grain, but actually a legume, alfalfa was originally grown in North Africa. It is now widely cultivated in various parts of the world. Over 27 million acres in America alone are devoted to alfalfa each year, and organically grown alfalfa seed is easily found in most natural foods stores.

Alfalfa sprouts are among the basic sprouts grown at the Ann Wigmore Foundation. Pound for pound, they are one of the most nutritious foods you can eat. The roots of mature alfalfa plants can reach several feet down into the soil, collecting hard-to-find trace elements as they go. Alfalfa sprouts are a good source of B-complex vitamins, along with vitamins A, C, E, and K. They also contain calcium, magnesium, potassium, iron, and the trace minerals selenium and zinc. If they are grown in indirect light, their nutritional content is further enhanced by the development of chlorophyll.

Alfalfa sprouts are among the most versatile. Use them to make salads, sandwiches, green drinks, soups, and sprout loaves.

Almonds are native to Persia, where they have been cultivated for hundreds of years. Most of the almonds grown in the United States come from California. Almonds and almond sprouts are basic components of the Living Food Lifestyle because they supply an extremely high-quality protein.

Of all the nuts, almonds are one of the easiest to digest, especially after twenty-four to forty-eight hours of sprouting. They are an excellent source of protein, calcium, potassium, phosphorus, magnesium, and fats. In addition, they contain B vitamins and vitamin E. Sprouted almonds have a crunchy texture. Use them in salad dressings, to make beverages, yogurt, cheeses, sprout loaves, breads, cereals, granola, and desserts.

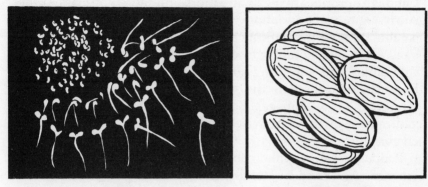

Alfalfa   Almonds

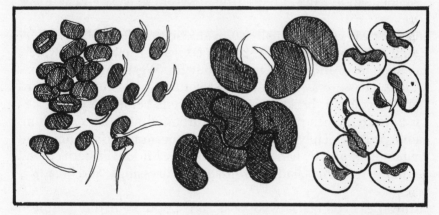

Adzuki Beans   Kidney Beans   Pinto Beans

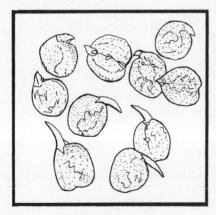
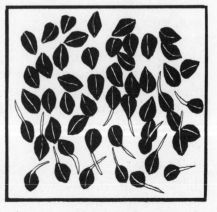

Chick Peas   Buckwheat

Cabbage sprouts are becoming more and more popular. At the Ann Wigmore Foundation we often sprout cabbage seeds in combination with others such as alfalfa, radish, and lentil. Cabbage and Chinese cabbage seeds are available from many seed companies and sprouting supply houses fairly inexpensively. In most cases, they are the same seeds used by gardeners and farmers to grow cabbages. So be sure the seeds you buy are organically grown. Otherwise you are likely to wind up with chemically treated seeds.

Cabbage sprouts, like cabbage itself, are a good source of vitamins A, C, and U, along with the trace elements iodine and sulfur. Use cabbage sprouts and cabbage sprout mixes in salads, sandwiches, green drinks, sprout loaves, and soups.

Chick peas were originally cultivated in the Middle East, where they are still considered a staple food item. They are also widely cultivated in India and throughout the Western Hemisphere. Chick peas are available at most natural foods stores. Discard any discolored, broken or chipped seeds before sprouting.

Sprouted chick peas are rich in carbohydrates, fiber, calcium, and protein. They also provide magnesium, potassium, and vitamins A and C. Use them to make the Middle Eastern spread hummus, and in salads, sprout loaves, dressings, and breads.

Cow peas, or black-eyed peas, are popular in the Southern United States. Cow peas are medium-sized white beans with black spots. Try to get organically grown beans if possible. If not, you can try sprouting the ones obtainable in the supermarket.

Cow peas, like most of the peas and some of the beans we use for sprouting, are a good source of protein, vitamins A and C, magnesium, and potassium. They are surprisingly flavorful sprouts that can be used in salads, marinates, sprout loaves, and green drinks.

Fenugreek is a small seed with a light tan color and a pleasant herb-like smell. Although fenugreek is a native of western Asia, most of the fenugreek seeds sold in this country come from northern Africa.

A valuable blood and kidney cleanser with a pungent flavor, fenugreek is an excellent source of phosphorus and iron. It contains a number of trace elements as well. Fenugreek is best sprouted with other seeds to mellow its flavor. Use mixtures containing fenugreek sprouts in salads, sprout loaves, and green drinks.

Lentils, which are native to Central Asia, are small beans with a round, flat shape. Use only green lentils for home sprouting, because red lentils are hulled after harvest, and most of the beans will not sprout. Organically grown lentils are available at most natural foods stores.

Lentil sprouts are rich in protein, iron, and vitamin C, and are one of the basic sprouts grown at the Ann Wigmore Foundation. Use them in salads with the sea vegetable dulse, in sprout loaves, in breads, and in green drinks. They also go well with marinated vegetables.

Mung beans, or Chinese bean sprouts, are another staple at the Foundation, and are second only to alfalfa in popularity for home growing. These sprouts have been used widely by people in the Far East for centuries. The small, green-colored seeds are available at most natural foods stores and Oriental groceries.

Mung sprouts are a good source of protein, especially the amino acid methionine, which may have a calming effect on the body. They are also rich in vitamin C, and contain healthful stores of the minerals iron and potassium. Use mung sprouts in salads, sandwiches, green drinks, soups, sprout loaves, and marinated vegetables.

Peas are a legume native to the Mediterranean. Green and yellow peas can be found in most natural foods stores, and in supermarkets. The ones you use for sprouting must be whole peas, as split peas won't sprout.

Peas are a good source of protein, carbohydrates, fiber, vitamin A, and several important minerals, including iron, potassium, and magnesium. Green peas also supply chlorophyll. Use sprouted peas to make dips, and in soups, sprout loaves, salads, and salad dressings.

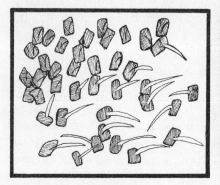

Fenugreek

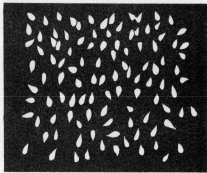

Sesame Seeds

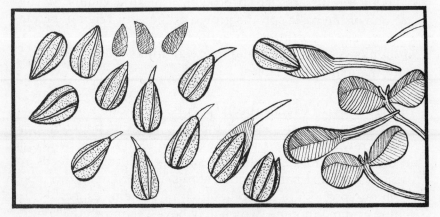

Sunflower Seeds

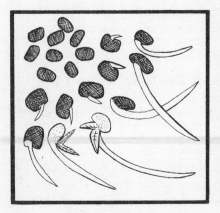

Mung Beans

Lentils

Pumpkin seeds are one of the more valuable seeds for the purpose of sprouting. The pumpkin seeds most often sold in stores are cultivated in the warmer climates of the world. The hulled seeds are larger than sunflower seeds and have a dark greenish color. Their flavor is also richer than that of sunflower seeds.

Pumpkin seeds contain high-quality proteins as well as fats, vitamin E, phosphorus, iron, and zinc (a trace element that is often lacking in the modern diet). As they are always used hulled, pumpkin seeds do not require long sprouting times; in fact, they are best when eaten after about twenty-four hours of sprouting. Use the sprouted seeds to make salad dressings, sprout loaves, yogurts, cheeses, desserts, snacks, and beverages.

Rye is native to western Asia and the Near East. Of all the cereal grasses, rye is the most hardy. You can find whole rye berries at many natural foods stores. They resemble wheatberries in size and shape, but are grey in color.

Sprouted rye is slightly sweet, indicating the presence of carbohydrates. It is also a good source of protein, B-complex vitamins, and vitamin E. The minerals phosphorus, potassium, and magnesium are found in sprouted rye as well. Try sprouting rye berries along with lentils and wheat for a tasty mix. Use sprouted rye to make cereals, and in salads, breads, granola, and milks.

Sesame seeds, which originally grew wild in India, were one of the first cultivated foods. Now they are grown in most parts of the world. Light and dark varieties are sold either hulled or unhulled. Purchase seeds with the hulls on (unhulled) for use in sprouting, because hulled seeds usually have been treated with harsh chemical solvents.

Sesame seeds are rich in protein, fats, the B vitamins, vitamin E, and fiber. They are a good source of several vital minerals as well, most notably magnesium, potassium, iron, phosphorus, and calcium. In fact, milk made from sprouted sesame seeds contains nearly as much calcium as cow's milk. Since the seeds are so small, they require only a short period of sprouting, usually one to three days. Sprouting them longer than this could cause them to take on a bitter flavor. Sesame sprouts are a basic component of Living Food nutrition. Use the sprouted seeds to make milks, cheeses, yogurts, salad dressings, breads, cereals, and candies.

Sunflower seeds were first used as food by the Indians of North and South America. Today, these versatile seeds are cultivated all over the world for food, oil, fabric, and dye. With their hulls removed, the seeds are small and grey in color. Hulled sunflower seeds for use in home sprouting are available at natural foods stores.

A staple of the Living Food program, sprouted sunflower seeds are one of the richest edible seeds. They are a good source of protein, fats, the B-complex vitamins, and vitamin E. In addition, they supply significant amounts of the minerals calcium, iron, phosphorus, potassium, and magnesium. Sunflower sprouts can be used to make delicious salad dressings, cheeses, milks, sprout loaves, breads, candies, and desserts. Sunflower *greens* (see Chapter 7) are also tasty and nutritious.

Vegetable seeds such as radish, kale, watercress, broccoli, mustard, and turnip are excellent for home sprouting. Cabbage (see page 32) is one of the most nutritious vegetable sprouts. Many vegetable seeds are available in pound lots through the mail. The vegetable seeds we use regularly at the Ann Wigmore Foundation are radish, mustard, and those seeds in the cabbage family. These are most often mixed with other seeds, particularly alfalfa, to make sprouting mixes, as some of them have a rather strong flavor by themselves.

In general, vegetable seeds contain a little more vitamins and minerals than the parent plant. Most of the vegetable seed sprouts mentioned above are good sources of vitamin C, vitamin A, and minerals, including trace minerals.

Wheat, the staple grain of the world, currently provides more calories and protein to the human race than any other food. It is one of the basic sprouts grown at the Foundation. Wheatberries for home sprouting are easy to come by, as almost every natural foods store sells them. Buy soft spring wheat for sprouting.

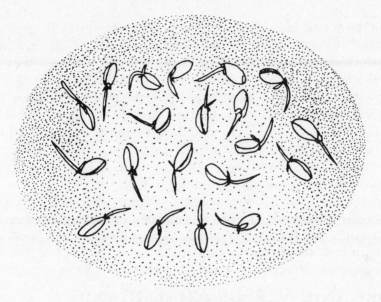

Wheat Sprouts

Sprouted wheat is an excellent source of protein, magnesium, phosphorus, B-complex vitamins, and vitamin E. It is also rich in energy-producing carbohydrates. Use sprouted wheat in salads, to make milks, and in desserts, breads, and cereals.

Of course, there are other seeds that can be sprouted and used for food. We have merely discussed the ones most commonly used for sprouting, and which for reasons of flavor and digestibility have become staples at the Ann Wigmore Foundation.

CHOOSING SEEDS FOR SPROUTING

When choosing seeds for sprouting, look for uniformity of shape, color, and perfection. Look at the seeds you wish to buy carefully. What you should see are thousands of distinct and perfect-looking seeds.

Broken, chipped or otherwise damaged seeds may lead to problems with rot or may not sprout at all. A handful of bad seeds will often spoil the bunch. Notice the color as well: are the red seeds, like adzuki, red; and the green ones, like mung, green? If the seeds are pink instead of red or lime green rather than deep green, they are probably not ripe and you should look for another source. Are there lots of sticks, stones, and dirt in with the seeds? You will have to separate all of this out, so be careful not to buy seeds that are loaded with rubble. Organically grown seeds will often look less clean and polished, but a quick wash before sprouting will remove any grime on them.

Buying bulk, unpackaged seeds in stores that stock them in bins will save you money and probably provide you with fresher seeds as well. In some cases organic seeds will be available only in bulk, as many growers don't have packaging machines and ship only by the fifty-pound bag. When possible buy in bulk for the best value.

ORGANIC VERSUS NONORGANIC

In a sense, all plants grown on soil are organic, but there are great differences in *how* they are grown. *Organically grown seeds* come from plants that are grown without the use of man-made chemical fertilizers, herbicides, and pesticides. They are balanced seeds grown on balanced soil. It is the very balance between the plant and the soil that protects it against disease, pests, and other dangers. Nonorganically grown seeds, on the other hand, usually come from plants that are grown on soil heavily fertilized with petrochemicals. The plants themselves are sprayed with a battery of harmful chemicals to ward off weeds and pests.

While some agricultural experts claim that the methods used to grow plants make no difference whatsoever, my experience has taught me otherwise. Every chemical agent affects the body in some way. Not only does petrochemical farming have the short-term effect of destroying our valuable topsoil, it also has a frightening potential to destroy our health. If you can obtain organically grown seeds for sprouting, it is well worth going out of your way to do so. At the same time that you safeguard your own health, you will support those growers who are attempting to enrich the soil and the health of human beings everywhere, rather than those who are depleting both.

6

Growing a Home Sprout Garden

Moisten your wheat, that the angel of water may enter it. Then set it in the air, that the angel of air may embrace it. And leave it from morning to evening beneath the sun, that the angel of sunshine may descend upon it.

Essene Gospel of Peace

Whereas growing an abundant vegetable garden in rich back-yard soil is beyond the reach of many people, growing a sprout garden indoors is simple, easy, and enjoyable. Variables such as fertilizers, weeds, killing frosts, and so on are not a concern for the kitchen gardener. And when you grow sprouts indoors, it is easy to provide them with just the right amounts of sun-light and water. If you follow the simple instructions in this chapter, very little can go wrong. You will be eating your first batch of fresh, home-grown sprouts one or two days after you set up your garden—you won't have to wait sixty to seventy days to see results. In fact, sprouting is so uncomplicated that in many homes the role of "chief family sprout grower" is given to one of the children.

There are several methods of home sprout growing—you may choose to set up your garden with jars, sprout bags, trays, and/or an automatic sprouter. Whatever method(s) you select, the basic steps are the same, from the initial soaking and drain-ing of the seeds, through the rinsing and care of the growing sprouts, to their eventual harvest and use as nutritious, health-ful food.

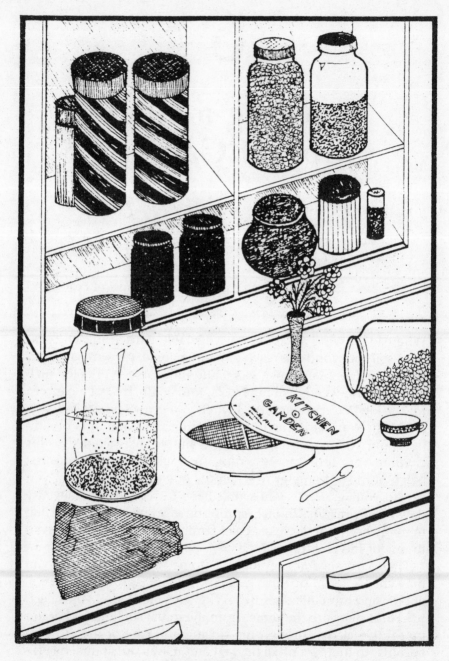

Sprouting Supplies

THE BASIC CARE OF SPROUTS

The basic care of sprouts focuses on keeping them moist while providing adequate drainage and air circulation. Find a good location for your sprout garden. A countertop near a sink is ideal, since you will need access to water and room for water to drain. Sprouts like to "get their feet wet" often, without being flooded with water. The more consistently you rinse and otherwise care for them, the healthier they will be. One reason that the sprouts grown in automatic sprout growers tend to come out uniformly good is that they are consistently rinsed and drained, without being handled too often (sprouts aren't crazy about being juggled around).

Like most plants, sprouts mature more quickly in warm weather, so soaking times should be monitored carefully and rinsing should be done more frequently to keep them cool. Keep your sprouts out of the direct reach of the afternoon sun during warm weather, as the combination of the heat indoors and the hot sun can literally cook the sprouts. Indirect light—a balance of sun and shade—is adequate for greening those sprouts that require light.

The chart on pages 56–59 summarizes the basic requirements of sprouts. With a little practice and some patience you will grow perfect sprouts with ease. If you do have a problem that isn't discussed in this chapter, write or call the Ann Wigmore Foundation.

WHAT TO SPROUT

At the Foundation in Boston, the basic sprouts grown are alfalfa, almonds, lentils, mung beans, sesame, sunflower, and wheat. Our experience has shown us that these are the easiest to grow, best-tasting, and most versatile. Other sprouts are grown on a more limited basis. Combinations of sprouts, with alfalfa as a base, are particularly popular.

In addition to the various sprouts, buckwheat and sunflower greens are grown at the Foundation, as is wheatgrass, a nutritious food that has healing qualities. Greens and wheatgrass are easy to grow indoors, especially once you have already set up a home sprout garden. Moreover, they are a delicious component of a healthful living foods diet. For these reasons, indoor gardening techniques for buckwheat and sunflower greens are discussed in Chapter 7 of this book. Detailed information about growing and using wheatgrass is available in *The Wheatgrass Book*.

GETTING STARTED

With ten half-gallon jars, or an automatic sprouter with three trays, and a variety of seeds, you can begin a home sprout garden that will supply you with enough sprouts to gain optimal nutrition at each meal. Try growing each of the basic sprouts. You will be able to make many of the recipes in Chapter 8 with them, and will experience a variety of flavors.

To start out using the jar method, get seven jars ready (keep the other three in reserve for later use). The table on the next page shows the amounts that are suggested for half-gallon jars.

If you are using an automatic sprout grower, merely spread the seeds evenly in different areas of the tray and watch them grow, harvesting each variety when it is ready to eat.

THE JAR METHOD

The jar method of home sprout growing is simple yet reliable. Wide-mouth glass jars are recommended, as you will need to fit your hand in them to remove the mature sprouts. Extensive testing at the Ann Wigmore Foundation has revealed that these jars are easy to work with and that they produce far better sprouts than plastic containers do. As mentioned above, ten half-gallon jars is a good number to have on hand.

In addition to the jars, you will need some pieces of cheesecloth, nylon mesh screening, or any other non-toxic material that will allow air to circulate. Use a piece of this material to cover each jar, and a string or rubber band to secure it. Make

Seven Jar Setup

Jar	Variety	Amount	Recipe Suggestions
1	almonds	1 cup	beverages, cheeses, salad dressings
2	alfalfa seeds	3–4 tablespoons	juices, salads, sprout loaves
3	lentils	1 cup	breads, juices, salads, sprout loaves
4	wheatberries	1 cup	breads, salads
5	mung beans (see page 48)	½ cup	juices, salads, sprout loaves
6	sunflower seeds (hulled)	1 cup	beverages, cheeses, salad dressings
	sesame seeds (unhulled)	1 cup	
7	alfalfa and multi-sprout mix (see page 53)	2–3 tablespoons alfalfa; other amounts will vary	salads

sure that this string or rubber band fits securely and that it will withstand heavy duty, or your sprouts could go flying everywhere.

Measure the appropriate amount of seed (see page 56) into the jar. Smaller seeds should just cover the bottom of the jar, while bigger seeds and beans should not fill the jar more than one-eighth to one-quarter full. Sprouts expand—for example, one pound of alfalfa seeds produces eight pounds of sprouts.

Cover the jar with the cheesecloth or screening. Then fill it halfway with water. Allow seeds to soak for the required length of time—approximately four to six hours for smaller seeds, and twelve hours for larger seeds and beans. After this time, drain off the water. Place the jar at a 45° angle, mouth down, in a place where it can drain freely. The small openings at the bottom will allow excess water to drain and air to circulate.

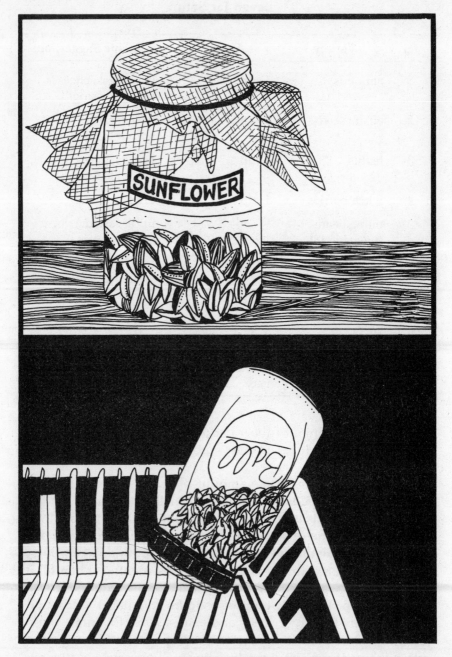

The Jar Method
Above: Soaking   Below: Draining

For best results, rinse the sprouts twice a day by placing the jar under the tap, filling it with water, and allowing it to overflow. As rinsing removes waste produced by the sprouts, the water coming out of the jar will appear a little foamy. After rinsing, replace the jar of sprouts at a 45° angle so that excess water will drain away. When the sprouts have matured, follow the procedures for harvesting and storage described later in this chapter.

USING SPROUT BAGS

Sprout bags are white, 8″ × 12″ drawstring bags made of special non-resinated nylon mesh screening. They are lightweight, highly durable, and machine-washable. Originally created for travel, these bags are relative newcomers to the sprouting scene. They can be ordered by mail and used to grow sprouts at home with results similar to those obtainable by the jar method. Ten sprout bags are all you need to start a home sprout garden; sprout bags are approximately equal in capacity to half-gallon jars.

To grow sprouts using this method, place the appropriate amount of seed in a sprout bag and place the bag in a bowl of water. Allow seeds to soak for the required length of time. After soaking, rinse the bag and hang it on the faucet or on a hook over the sink to drain for a couple of minutes. Then place the sprout bag inside a plastic bag with a few holes punched in it for ventilation, and hang to drain as before.

As in the jar method, rinse the sprouts twice a day. Simply remove the plastic bag and either dip the sprout bag in a bowl of water or rinse it under the faucet. Each time you rinse the sprouts, make sure to drain them thoroughly before putting the sprout bag back inside the plastic bag and hanging it up again.

To harvest the mature sprouts, follow the standard procedures described later in this chapter. Before starting a new batch of sprouts, wash the sprout bags with mild soap and soak them in clear water. The same basic procedures apply for traveling with sprout bags; additional hints for growing and transporting sprouts will be found in Chapter 9.

TRAY–TYPE SPROUTERS

Tray-type sprouters may be used to grow alfalfa sprouts and mixes of sprouts with alfalfa as the main ingredient. Alfalfa sprouts are especially suited to tray-type growers, as their leaves become green and they spread out like a carpet after five days of growth. These sprouts grow straighter than in jars as well.

The tray method has become the most popular way for commercial producers to grow alfalfa sprouts, as the finished produce is easier to store, stack, and display in markets. Their large tray-type growers are fully automated.

Small tray-type sprouters manufactured specifically for home use work well. The tray-type sprouters sold at natural food stores come with instructions and a cover, but are usually quite small (about twelve to fourteen inches in diameter). If you decide to buy these, you will need at least two to begin with.

Before we began using automatic sprouters at the Ann Wigmore Foundation, we used large plastic trays (approximately 24″ × 24″, and 2″ to 4″ deep) purchased from a nursery supply store. Trays about 10″ × 14″ are good for home use. For best results, get trays with holes that are a quarter of an inch in diameter or smaller. The bottoms of trays with larger holes can be covered with a sheet of nylon mesh screening. You will need a stiff vegetable brush to clean the tray and the mesh, as the tiny alfalfa sprout roots tend to get stuck in the holes.

If you are using one of the store-bought tray-type sprouters, follow the directions that come with it. Otherwise, use the following method to sprout seeds in a tray. Measure the amount of alfalfa seed or seed mix needed. (Use the same seed amounts as you would for a half-gallon size jar.) Soak the seeds for the specified amount of time in a jar of water. If the holes in the tray are small, you can either put the soaked seeds directly on the tray, or grow them in a jar for three days following the standard jar method. If the tray has holes greater than a quarter of an inch in diameter, it is best to start the seeds in a jar.

After the sprouts are one-quarter to one-half inch in length, spread them out in the bottom of the tray and place the entire tray inside a clear plastic bag. Punch a few holes in the plastic to let air circulate. Like the cover on a store-bought tray-type sprouter, the plastic bag will prevent the sprouts from drying out. Also try to keep the bottom of the tray slightly elevated, using a rack of some sort to allow air to reach the roots. Many of the store-bought tray-type sprouters are designed with small legs that facilitate air circulation.

Whether the sprouts are started in a jar or a tray, you will have to water them at least twice a day. There are two good ways to water trays. After removing the plastic, you can either mist the tray heavily with water from a clean spray bottle, or dip the whole tray in a bath of cool water, covering the sprouts.

On the fourth day the leaves of alfalfa sprouts will begin to turn green, and they will be ready to harvest a day or two later. Follow the standard harvesting and storage procedure described on pages 49–51.

SPROUTING AUTOMATICALLY

Automatic sprouters are the perfect solution for the person who wants an abundant supply of sprouts with a minimal amount of work. I have been using automatic sprouters for years, and I'm totally convinced of their overall effectiveness and reliability. One important advantage of this method is that you needn't tie up the kitchen countertop, as the sprouter can be placed almost anywhere there is light, a water pipe, and a drain or bucket to catch the rinse water. The unit comes with a self-tapping fitting for do-it-yourself installation.

The most popular style of automatic sprouter looks like a miniature chest of drawers with anywhere from two to ten stainless steel or plastic drawers. Each drawer is actually a tray set at an angle for proper drainage. A series of fine misters are suspended from pipes above each drawer. Usually the top drawer is covered with clear plastic, allowing light to reach the sprouts growing in it. Sprouts that do not require light, such as beans and grains, are grown in the lower drawers, which remain dark.

To use the sprouter, hook it up to water and power as directed in the manufacturer's instructions. Evenly sprinkle the appropriate amount of seeds into the tray (follow the growing instructions that come with the unit, as sizes of the growing areas vary in each), and turn it on. The sprouts will be misted every couple of hours and the excess water will be drained off. If your unit has three trays, harvest the top tray every four or five days. Move the next tray in line to the top position, wash the empty tray, and begin a new batch of sprouts. An optional "grow light" bulb can be placed over the top tray for greening the sprouts more quickly.

Without a doubt this is the most convenient and simple method of sprouting. Whereas sprouting in jars or bags is more cumbersome, time-consuming, and apt to be neglected, once a family decides to purchase an automatic grower they tend to use it regularly.

GROWING MUNG AND ADZUKI BEANS

Mung or Chinese bean sprouts and adzuki bean sprouts taste best when they are grown away from light and under pressure. Exposure to light tends to make them tougher, as the process of photosynthesis stimulates the development of cellulose as well as chlorophyll in the growing sprouts. When you finish reading this section you will know how professionals grow the beautiful bean sprouts sold in supermarkets.

To begin you will need a cylindrical container that is about ten to twelve inches deep and ten to fourteen inches in diameter. It should be made from stainless steel. (Do not use aluminum, as it is chemically reactive.) Punch or drill holes, three-sixteenths of an inch in diameter, at one- to two-inch intervals all around the container, including some on the bottom.

You will also need a plate (or another cover) that fits down inside the container, and a weight that will press down on the cover. A clean masonry brick will work well as a weight. This setup will keep light out and force the sprouts to push against each other and against the weight as they grow, making them thicker and more juicy.

You will need one or two cups of raw, unsprouted mung or adzuki beans for a container of the size described above. Soak the beans in a jar of water for twelve hours. Then pour off the water, rinse the beans, and place them in the stainless steel container. Put the plate on top, but do not add the weight at this time.

You will also need a dark-colored plastic container a little bit larger than the stainless steel one, to help keep out any light. Place some stones or a wire rack in the bottom of the plastic container; then set the stainless steel container on top (it should fit completely inside the plastic container). The stones or rack will allow air to circulate and prevent excess water from damaging the bottom layer of sprouts.

In the morning and the evening, take out the stainless steel container, remove the plate, and rinse the sprouts under cold water for about two minutes. Then let the water drain out of the holes for a few seconds before replacing the plate and putting the container back inside the plastic one.

On the third day of sprouting, place the weight on top of the plate. Continue to rinse the sprouts twice a day for another four to five days, or until they are large and plump. If you encounter a problem with spoilage, try rinsing the sprouts more frequently, making sure that the water you use is cold. If this does not help, try purchasing another batch of bean seeds.

If you visit the Foundation, either as a two-week guest or during the weekly open house, you can see all of the different sprouting methods in operation.

HARVESTING YOUR SPROUTS

Harvesting is the process whereby you gather the mature sprouts. In harvesting certain sprouts, it is generally necessary to remove and discard the indigestible hulls. Adzuki, alfalfa, cabbage, clover, fenugreek, mung, and radish taste better with their hulls removed (hulled). In addition, these sprouts will store much longer in the refrigerator without their hulls. If, however, you are growing them for the sole purpose of juicing, the sprouts, hulls and all, can be run through the juicer. (The indigestible hulls of sunflower seeds should be removed *before* sprouting.)

Lentils, peas, and grains do not need to be hulled before eating or storage. To do so would be difficult anyway, as their hulls are soft and do not readily detach from the seeds. Tray-

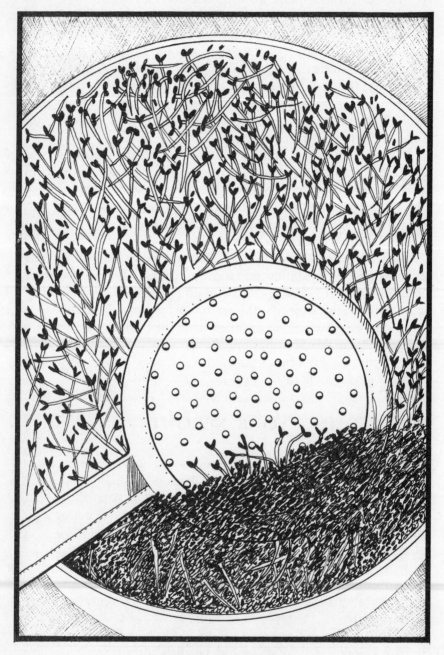

**Harvesting Your Sprouts
Rinsing off the hulls.**

type sprouters, and light, aid the hulling of alfalfa sprouts, as the leaves will open wider, casting off their hulls.

To hull sprouts, place them in the sink and fill it halfway with cool water. Agitate the sprouts gently with your fingers to loosen the hulls. Most of the hulls will rise to the surface, while some will sink to the bottom. Push the ones that float to one corner of the sink. Scoop them off the surface and compost or discard them. Using both hands, with fingers spread apart, gently reach underneath the hulled sprouts and scoop them out of the water. Try not to stir up the hulls on the bottom. Place the sprouts in a colander to drain before using them.

Transfer unused sprouts to a clean glass jar with a cover or a sealable plastic bag, and store them in the refrigerator. Sprouts that are hulled, drained well, and stored in glass or plastic will keep from seven to ten days in the refrigerator, growing slowly until you decide to use them.

WHAT HAPPENS IF . . .

Home sprout growing is generally simple and trouble-free. Nevertheless, as you get involved in the sprouting process, questions and problems are bound to arise. A batch of sprouts may mysteriously spoil, practically overnight. Or you may forget to attend to them and wonder if they can be salvaged. Most of the time you will find that you can solve the problem yourself with a little common-sense reasoning. A few hints on troubleshooting may help you, too.

The most frequent problem encountered in the sprouting process is spoilage. Bad seeds, inconsistent rinsings or too much heat, contaminated water, and inadequate ventilation are the most common causes of spoilage. Spoiled sprouts do not taste good, and can quickly contaminate healthy sprouts. Equally important, they have lost much of their nutritional value.

If you are careful to remove cracked or broken seeds from the batch before sprouting, you will minimize the risk of spoilage. Also, if upon filling the jar with water for soaking, you notice any small insects floating to the surface of the water, dispose of that batch of seeds—not just the jarful, but any other seeds you may have stored them with. It is best to store each type of raw, unsprouted seed in its own glass or plastic container with a cover, to prevent insects in one batch from contaminating others. The most common insect pests are weevils, which do their damage by attacking the germ of the seeds. While the damage isn't visible, the seed will sprout half-spoiled. So watch for insects.

Another problem you may encounter upon occasion is discovering an occasional "hard" seed in with your harvested sprouts. Hard seeds are seeds that refuse to sprout. They are nature's insurance against extreme weather conditions such as flood or drought. Even if most of the seeds produced by the plant are wiped out, there are always some hard seeds that will not begin germinating immediately, but will do so later, when conditions are more favorable.

The number of hard seeds per pound varies greatly. And there is no way to identify them just by looking. They look like the other seeds, but remain hard as a rock. Even so, hard seeds are rare. If you ever get a batch of seeds with an unusual number of hard seeds, replace the seeds with others from a different store or supplier.

A potential problem, unrelated to the quality of the seeds, is the temperature of the sprouting environment. If it gets hot outside (and inside) put a fan in the room to circulate the air, and rinse the sprouts more often—every four or five hours during the day, if necessary. If you are using an automatic sprout grower, be sure to tap into the cold water and not the hot.

Another factor that can contribute to spoilage is the contamination of the water used to soak the seeds. When you soak seeds in "bad" water, they can be attacked by certain microbes that cause them to grow half-spoiled. If you are sure the seeds are good—you have grown other batches with the same seed— and the room isn't too hot, try filtering the water used for soaking the seeds, or soak them in pure spring water. Adding a little powdered kelp and wheatgrass to the water used for soaking might also help by providing trace minerals and nutrients for the seeds.

If the sprouts you harvest taste bitter, or have an unpleasant texture or aroma, make sure that you neither drown the next batch of seeds with excessive soaking nor grow the sprouts too long. In the case of mung or adzuki beans, make sure not to expose them to light; except when they are grown in sprout mixtures, they should be kept in the dark.

Inadequate ventilation may also contribute to spoilage during the sprouting process. At times, some of the sprouts in a jar or tray will go bad. These are usually located at the neck of the jar or the bottom of the tray, where there is less air circulation. If the rest of the sprouts are unaffected, merely remove the spoiled sprouts, wash the others well in cool water, and either continue sprouting them or harvest and store them.

Upon occasion, harvested sprouts may spoil in storage. Generally this happens when a few sprouts sitting in a little pool of water in the bottom of the storage container begin to decompose. If this happens, merely remove any spoiled sprouts that you see, and wash the others well. They should be fine as long as you do not wait too long to eat them.

The sprouting chart on pages 56–59 details the recommended times for soaking the various seeds and growing the mature sprouts. If you follow these recommendations carefully, your home sprout garden should not present you with any unconquerable problems.

MIXING SPROUTS HARMONIOUSLY

Although different sprouts can be combined in a salad after they have been grown separately in individual containers, they can also be grown together for convenience. There are two general rules for mixing harmonious combinations of sprouts. First, use seeds that have similar rates of growth. Second, consider the flavor of the seeds when determining their proportions in the mix.

When creating your own combinations of seeds to sprout, you will need to use a little common sense. If a seed takes only two days to mature, it is best to mix it with other seeds that mature in two to three days. Likewise, sprouts such as alfalfa, radish, mung, and others that take long to mature should be mixed together. Some sprouts, including sunflower, lentil, wheat, chick pea, and cow pea, can be eaten either long or

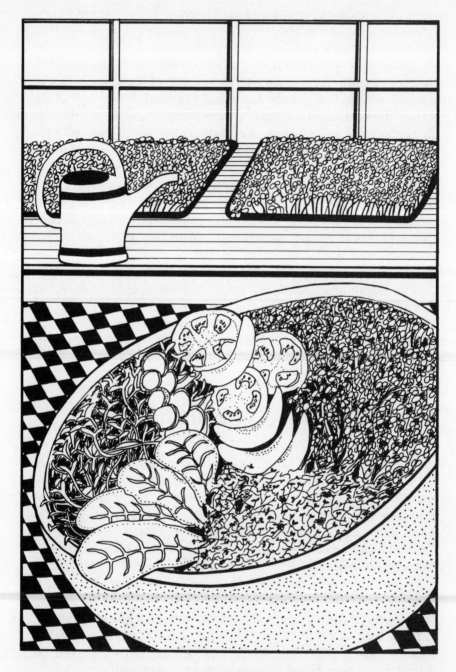

Sprouts and greens are easy to grow.

short, and are therefore easily combined either with shorter- or longer-growing seeds.

Also, use the flavor of each seed to determine how much to sprout in comparison to the others. For example, pungent radish, fenugreek, or mustard seeds are best mixed with at least 80 percent alfalfa or other mild-tasting sprouts.

Use the same sprouting methods to grow combinations of seeds that you use to grow single varieties. With practice you will be able to approximate the desired measurements by eye. To start out with, here are a few of the favorite combinations used at the Ann Wigmore Foundation, listed according to their uses.

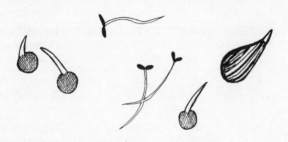

Sprout Combinations

Breads and Cereals

Wheat 50%, Chick pea 50%
Wheat 50%, Lentil 50%
Wheat 50%, Rye 50%
Wheat 50%, Sunflower 50%
Wheat 33%, Almond 33%, Sunflower 33%

Soups, Salads, and Juices

Alfalfa 60%, Lentil 25%, Wheat 15%
Alfalfa 60%, Cabbage 20%, Sunflower 20%
Alfalfa 50%, Cabbage 10%, Lentil 10%, Mung 10%, Radish 10%, Rye 10%
Lentil 50%, Adzuki 25%, Chick pea 25%
Lentil 40%, Mung 40%, Cow pea 20%
Mung 25%, Lentil 25%, Sunflower 25%, Wheat 25%

SPROUTING CHART

Variety	Soak (hours)	Dry Measure*	Length at Harvest	Ready in (days)	Sprouting Tips
Adzuki	12	1 cup	½"–1"	3–5	Easy sprouter. Try short & long.
Alfalfa	4–6	3–4 table-spoons	1"–1½"	4–6	Place in light to develop chloro-phyll 1–2 days before harvest.
Almond	12	1 cup	0"	1	Swells up, does not sprout.
Cabbage	4–6	⅓ cup	1"	4–5	Develops chlorophyll when mature.
Chick Pea	12	1 cup	½"	2–3	Mix with lentils & wheat, or use alone.
Clover	4–6	3 table-spoons	1"–1½"	4–5	Mix with other seeds. Develops chlorophyll.
Corn	12	1 cup	½"	2–3	Use sweet corn. Try short & long.
Cow Pea	12	1 cup	½"–1"	3–6	Grow in dark. Try short & medium.
Fenugreek	8	½ cup	½"–1"	3–5	Pungent flavor; mix with other seeds.
Green Pea	12	1 cup	½"	2–3	Use whole peas.
Lentil	12	1 cup	¼"–¾"	3–5	Earthy flavor. Try short & long. Versatile sprout.
Millet	8	1 cup	¼"	2–3	Use unhulled type.

*per half-gallon jar

Nutritional Highlights	Suggested Uses
high-quality protein; iron, vitamin C	casseroles, Oriental dishes, salads, sandwiches, sprout loaves
vitamins A, B, C, E, & K; rich in minerals and trace elements	juices, salads, sandwiches, soups, sprout loaves
rich in protein, fats, minerals, vitamins B & E	breads, cheeses, desserts, dressings, milks
vitamins A, C, & U; trace elements	cole slaw, salads, sandwiches, soups
carbohydrates, fiber, protein, minerals	breads, casseroles, dips, salads, spreads, sprout loaves
vitamins A & C; trace elements	breads, salads, sandwiches, soups
carbohydrates, fiber, minerals, vitamins A, B, & E	breads, cereals, grain dishes, granola, snacks
protein, vitamins A & C, minerals	Oriental dishes, salads, sprout loaves
rich in iron, phosphorus, trace elements	casseroles, curries, juices, salads, soups, sprout loaves
carbohydrates, fiber, protein, minerals, vitamins A & C	casseroles, dips, dressings, salads, soups, sprout loaves
rich in protein, iron and other minerals, vitamin C	breads, casseroles, curries, marinated vegetables, salads, soups, spreads, sprout loaves
carbohydrates, fiber, vitamins B & E, protein	breads, casseroles, cereals, salads, soups

SPROUTING CHART—*Continued*

Variety	Soak (hours)	Dry Measure*	Length at Harvest	Ready in (days)	Sprouting Tips
Mung	12	½ cup	½″–1½″	3–6	Grow in dark. Rinse in cold water for 1 minute.
Mustard	4–6	¼ cup	1″	4–5	Hot flavor; mix with other seeds.
Oats	12	1 cup	¼″–½″	2–3	Find whole sprouting type.
Pumpkin	8	1 cup	0″	1	Swells up, does not sprout.
Radish	4–6	¼ cup	1″	4–5	Hot flavor; mix with other seeds. Develops chlorophyll.
Rye	12	1 cup	¼″–½″	2–3	Try mixing with wheat & lentils.
Sesame	4–6	1 cup	0″	1–2	Tiny sprout, turns bitter if left too long.
Sunflower	8	2 cups	0″–½″	1–3	Use hulled seeds. Mix with alfalfa & grow 4–5 days.
Triticale	12	1 cup	¼″–½″	2–3	A grain hybrid like wheat.
Water-cress	4–6	4 table-spoons	½″	4–5	Spicy; mix with other seeds.
Wheat	12	1 cup	¼″–½″	2–3	Try short & long. For sweeter taste, mix with other seeds.

*per half-gallon jar

Nutritional Highlights	Suggested Uses
high-quality protein; iron, potassium, vitamin C	juices, Oriental dishes, salads, sandwiches, soups, sprout loaves
mustard oil, vitamins A & C, minerals	juices, salads, sandwiches, soups
vitamins B & E, protein, carbohydrates, fiber, minerals	breads, casseroles, cereals, soups, sprout loaves
protein, fats, vitamin E, phosphorus, iron, zinc	breads, cereals, cheeses, desserts, dressings, milks, snacks, sprout loaves, yogurts
potassium, vitamin C	dressings, juices, Mexican-style food, salads, sandwiches, soups
vitamins B & E, minerals, protein, carbohydrates	breads, cereals, granola, milks, salads, soups
rich in protein, calcium and other minerals; vitamins B & E, fats, fiber	breads, candies, cereals, cheeses, dressings, milks, salads, yogurts
rich in minerals, fats, protein, vitamins B & E	breads, cereals, cheeses, desserts, dressings, milks, salads, soups, sprout loaves, yogurts
see wheat	*see* wheat
vitamins A & C, minerals	breads, garnishes, salads, sandwiches
carbohydrates, protein, vitamins B & E, phosphorus	breads, cereals, desserts, granola, milks, salads, snacks, soups

7

Growing Greens Indoors

To own a bit of ground, to scratch it with a hoe, to plant seeds, and watch the renewal of life—this is the commonest delight of the race, the most satisfactory thing a man can do.

Charles Dudley Warner

Freshly grown sunflower greens and buckwheat lettuce are a tasty part of a healthful diet. In contrast to sprouts, which require no longer than five or six days to grow and do not require the use of soil, these indoor greens are grown on an inch of soil for about seven days. Nutritionally and flavorwise, they can replace more expensive lettuce and salad greens.

There is nothing difficult about growing your own fresh salad greens indoors, especially if you are already growing sprouts. However, growing greens does require some different techniques and equipment. These differences are the focus of this chapter.

At the Foundation in Boston, we have created an indoor gardening system for growing buckwheat lettuce and sunflower greens. You will find that the Living Food indoor gardening system is virtually self-sufficient. It requires little time and effort—and no costly supplies. The first difference from sprout gardening is that you should buy sunflower seeds that have *not* had their hulls removed (unhulled, as opposed to hulled). The buckwheat seeds that you purchase should also be unhulled. Both types are sprouted in jars for a day. They are subsequently placed on an inch of soil and watered. Then they are covered to keep light out for three days. On the fourth day, the cover is removed and the tray is placed in indirect light. The greens are watered daily until harvest time. For information about growing wheatgrass (a versatile and nutritious food with healing properties) in your indoor garden, see *The Wheatgrass Book*.

ABOUT BUCKWHEAT LETTUCE AND SUNFLOWER GREENS

Buckwheat is a plant with small, dark seeds that are somewhat triangular in shape. It is cultivated for use as a grain in the Northeast and North Central parts of the United States, and in various other places around the world. I have been growing buckwheat lettuce (greens) in my indoor garden for years, primarily for use in salads. Seven-day-old buckwheat lettuce has rich red stems and round, deep green leaves. These greens are an excellent source of chlorophyll, vitamins A and C, calcium, and lecithin (a fatty substance that is valuable in the diet because it helps the body to eliminate excess cholesterol). Buckwheat lettuce can also be used in making juices and soups.

The unhulled, black and white striped sunflower seeds obtainable in health food stores can, under favorable conditions, quickly grow into mature plants, ultimately producing the golden-yellow sunflowers that are a familiar sight in the countryside. While the seven-day-old sunflower plant may have a less striking appearance than the cheerful sunflower swaying on its long stalk, it is remarkably suitable for use as a salad green. Seven-day-old sunflower greens contain the various nutrients found in sunflower sprouts (see page 36), with the added benefit of chlorophyll. Along with buckwheat lettuce, these greens have been a mainstay of the Living Food Lifestyle for a number of years. They also can be used in blending soups.

SETTING UP AN INDOOR GARDEN

The first step in setting up your own indoor garden system will be finding a location to plant and store the trays of greens. You will also need a place to keep seeds and topsoil or compost. Since I live on the third floor of our Boston Foundation, I both plant and store all my supplies right in my kitchen. If you live in a house you may want to set up the system in the basement, in the garage, on the back porch, or, as I have done, in the kitchen. You may also choose to divide up the operations, for example, by storing soil and actually doing the planting in the basement, setting trays in upstairs windows, or soaking seeds in jars by the kitchen sink. Whatever setup you choose, though, you will need plenty of indirect sunlight for the growing plants and a warm place to start the trays off during the winter months (65–75° F is ideal).

GROWING GREENS INDOORS

If you use the method that I recommend, you will need to seek out some good topsoil and some peat moss, or a mixture of topsoil and compost (see page 69). Topsoil is the first twelve to twenty inches of dark-colored soil immediately beneath the grass on your lawn, or under the leaves covering the surface of a wooded area. If you live in a city, don't start digging up the public park—take a drive to the suburbs to get some topsoil, or buy it in large bags from a florist or garden supply store.

When taking topsoil from a wooded area, especially where pine trees are growing, mix about a half pint of ground limestone (lime) into a trash barrel full of soil. This will offset the acidity of the soil and make your indoor greens richer-tasting and easier to grow. Lime is inexpensive, and is available at any garden center. Ordinary lawn topsoil does not usually need lime, but you may add a handful or two per barrelful of soil just to be on the safe side. If you aren't mixing compost into the soil, mix the soil with peat moss (which is available at garden shops) in a 75–25 ratio. If you are using compost from an outdoor garden, it should be screened to remove large stones, sticks, and other debris, before being mixed with the topsoil. Do not use compost that has been treated with animal manures, as it may contain harmful bacteria.

To produce one tray of buckwheat lettuce and another of sunflower greens per day you will need to start off with at least two barrels full of topsoil and half a bale of peat moss. Along with this you will need two additional empty barrels to begin composting the used plant mats. Four barrels, two of which are

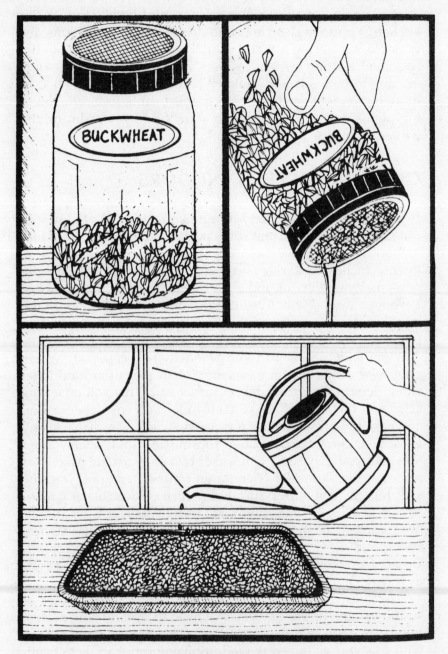

Growing Buckwheat Greens
Soaking, draining, and planting the seeds.

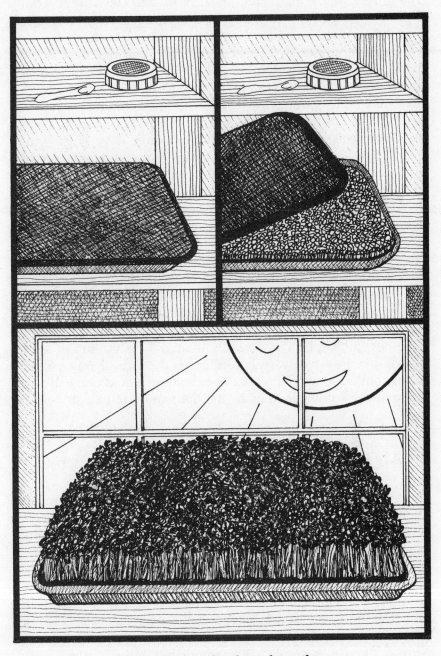

**Cover the tray for three days, then
uncover and set in indirect light.**

full of soil, and a half bale of peat moss will take care of your soil needs for a few weeks. After that time you will be able to use the recycled soil mats from the compost barrels.

For planting seeds, I recommend that you purchase some hard plastic trays. Restaurant supply stores will often sell you cafeteria trays about 10" × 14" in size. Unlike the nursery trays that may be used for growing sprouts, these trays are shallow and should not have any holes in them. You will need one tray to cover each planted tray for the first three days of growth. Start with about ten trays if you plan to harvest one tray of greens per day. Fifteen trays will enable you to produce one tray of buckwheat and one of sunflower per day.

To soak sunflower and buckwheat seeds, you will need some wide-mouth jars. While the seeds are soaking and sprouting, cover the jars with squares of nylon mesh screening and a rubber band (as described in Chapter 6).

Besides water and a little patience, the only other thing you will need is seeds. When purchasing buckwheat or sunflower seeds to grow for greens, buy them with their hulls on, or "unhulled." If possible, obtain organically grown seeds; they are sure not to have been chemically treated. The amount of seed to use per tray will vary according to the size of tray you're using, but three-quarters of a cup of sunflower and one-half cup of buckwheat will generally be the right amount for a 10" × 14" tray.

PLANTING INSTRUCTIONS

Before planting, wash the seeds to remove any grime or dust. Next, place them in the jar and fill it with water. Put a screen over the top and let it sit overnight (or for twelve hours). Drain the seeds after soaking, rinse them well, and let them sprout in the jar at a 45° angle for another twelve hours.

After the seeds have sprouted for twelve hours, spread a one-inch layer of soil at the bottom of the tray and smooth it out, leaving small trenches around the edges to catch excess water. Pour the sprouted seeds in the middle of the tray and spread them out evenly with your hands, covering the soil. Ideally, each seed should touch the next, without being piled on top of any other. Sprinkle the tray with water, making it damp (but not swampy), and cover it with another tray.

The second tray, used as a cover, acts as a mini-greenhouse that keeps moisture and heat in, and light out of, the growing environment. After you have watered and covered the tray, set it aside for three days.

At the end of three days uncover the tray, water it well, and place it in indirect light. The more light the plants get the larger and thicker the leaves will be, whereas too little light will produce tall, leggy plants with tiny leaves. A good balance of indirect sunlight and shade will produce greens that are thick and juicy.

If you uncover a tray and see greenish-blue mold instead of baby plants, you may have used poor-quality seeds, or drowned good seeds by over-soaking. It is also possible that you may have over-watered the tray after planting. Try again with new seeds and less water, and make sure that the spot where you put the tray is not too warm. It should be between 65° and 75° F.

Once the greens are set out in the light, they will need to be watered every day or every other day depending on the weather, humidity, and indoor temperature. The first or second time you water the plants, mix a tablespoon of powdered kelp into the water to add trace elements and iodine that will be taken up by the plants. Try not to muddy the soil, but keep it moist at all times. If by accident a tray is allowed to dry out, resist the temptation to flood it with water, as this will only shock the plants further. Instead moisten the soil, and make sure it doesn't dry out again for the next few days. Don't worry if the plants refuse to stand up straight again. Drooping is caused by the lack of water, and the greens will be good to eat anyway.

After about a week, the greens will be about five to eight inches tall and ready to harvest. In cooler weather it may take a little longer for them to fully mature, whereas during hot summer weather they can reach ten inches in five days. The chart on pages 68-69 summarizes the basic requirements of indoor garden greens.

To harvest buckwheat lettuce and sunflower greens, cut as close as possible to the soil without pulling any up with the plants. Many nutrients are concentrated close to the soil. A

INDOOR GARDENING CHART

Variety	Soak (hours)	Dry Measure*	Sprouting Time (hours)	Length at Harvest	Ready in (days)
Buckwheat	12	½ cup	12	5″–8″	7
Sunflower	12	¾ cup	12	5″–8″	7

*per 10″ × 14″ tray

sharp knife and a sawing action will cut easily. If some soil does come up with the plants, merely rinse the root ends with plain water before juicing or eating the greens. Do not rinse the plants if you are going to store them, however, as the water speeds their decomposition. Buckwheat and sunflower greens will last seven to ten days in the refrigerator. Nevertheless, the fresher they are the better-tasting they will be, and the more nutritious as well.

Planting Check List

As a handy reference to growing indoor garden greens, here is a summary of the steps we have just discussed:

- Mix 2 or 3 barrels of topsoil 75–25 with peat moss or 50–50 screened compost. Obtain 10 to 15 hard plastic cafeteria trays, several wide-mouth jars, and buckwheat and sunflower seeds with their hulls still on.

- Wash seeds and soak them for 12 hours; then allow them to sprout for 12 hours.

- On trays, spread soil 1 inch deep, leaving shallow trenches at the edges to catch excess water. Smooth the soil and spread the sprouted seeds on top.

- Water the planted tray, cover with another tray, and set aside for 3 days.

Nutritional Highlights	Suggested Uses
chlorophyll, vitamins A & C, calcium, lecithin	juices, salads, soups
chlorophyll, vitamins A & C, minerals	juices, salads, soups

- On the fourth day, uncover the tray, water it, and set it in indirect light. Continue watering the tray daily or every other day, as needed, to keep it moist.

- Harvest plants with a sharp knife when they reach 7–10 inches in height, cutting as close to the roots as possible without pulling up clumps of soil. Use greens as soon after harvesting as possible, and store unused portions in a sealable plastic or glass container in the refrigerator.

RECLAIMING TOPSOIL THROUGH COMPOSTING

After you harvest greens, you will be left with a mat of roots and short stems that can easily be recycled to make new soil for planting in a few weeks. This recycling process is called composting.

Composting is nature's way of building and maintaining the fertility of the soil. In the forest fallen leaves and dead branches cover the earth, making rich compost for the trees that continue to grow. In fact, everything that has been taken from the soil to nourish growing plants must be returned to it through decomposition of plant and animal matter if it is to continue to support new growth. Compost is a mixture of soil and plant residues that are decomposed into a rich humus by the action of worms, microorganisms, and enzymes in the soil.

The modern growing techniques used by agribusiness farmers often neglect to replace the trace minerals and organic matter that crops take out of the soil as they grow. Sometimes an attempt is made to replenish some of these vital elements by the use of synthetic chemical fertilizers. Unfortunately, there is no food in synthetic chemical fertilizers to support the continuation of soil enzymes, worms, and microorganisms that live on organic matter—and after a few years of agricultural exploitation, the soil becomes a useless desert, barely able to grow weeds. Acres upon acres of land all over the world are being ruined in this way every year.

Composting is one solution to the problem of soil depletion. It is a way of reclaiming poor soil and restoring natural balance to the topsoil. In the presence of organic matter, soil enzymes and organisms like the friendly earthworm thrive and multiply, enriching the soil and feeding the plants grown on it with top-quality plant nutrients. This is precisely the way nature has preserved plant life on earth for centuries. And on a large scale, it's the only way we can ensure that the soil will be fertile enough to produce food for our children—and theirs.

An important worker in your home compost pile is the earthworm, whose job it is to digest organic matter and convert it into rich plant nutrients. Earthworms leave behind castings that are an extremely valuable source of nitrogen, minerals, and other nutrients. The castings contain five times the nitrogen, seven times the phosphate, and eleven times the potassium of ordinary topsoil.

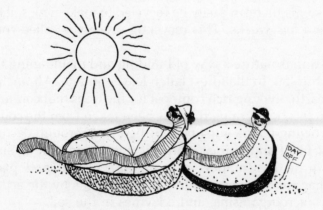

You can obtain earthworms from a compost pile or an old pile of leaves, or you can buy some at any bait and tackle shop. Ask for red wigglers. Add at least a couple of handfuls to your compost; nature will take care of the rest. The earthworms will go to work producing their weight in castings every twenty-four hours.

COMPOSTING INSTRUCTIONS

To start your home composting system you will need two empty barrels with lids. Drill holes spaced at two-inch intervals all around each barrel, including a few in the bottom. Place a shallow container of some sort underneath each barrel to serve as a drainage tray. Inverted flat trash can lids work well. It is best if the barrel is supported an inch or two off the container, to allow air circulation underneath. A couple of bricks will do nicely.

When you harvest some greens, break up the mats into pieces and place them in a layer in the bottom of the barrel. On top of this layer, spread some vegetable scraps or pulp that has been ejected from your juicer. Following the scraps, put in the earthworms, and cover them with another layer of broken-up mats. (Do *not* use fruit scraps, as they can cause excessive leakage in your compost barrel. Store vegetable scraps and pulp in a sealed container until you have enough mats to cover them.) As you harvest mats, repeat this layering technique, only without adding any more earthworms, until the barrel is full. After each layer is placed in the barrel, cover it with a lid. Also mix in a handful of lime per barrel to keep the soil slightly alkaline.

When the compost barrel is full, the decomposition of the mats and vegetable matter intensifies. As long as the barrels are in a warm place, but out of direct sunlight, the compost will develop into rich soil, ready for use in two to three months. If you want to use your compost sooner, in one to two months, remove the lid every week and stir up the contents of the barrel with a shovel. This will expose the contents to more oxygen, speeding up the rate of decomposition.

You will know when the compost is ready by scooping out a shovelful and examining it. If it is crumbly, dark, and without any bad odor or trace of scraps, it is ready. To use the new compost for planting, mix it with 25 percent peat moss.

Compost barrels can be kept in the basement, in a back hallway, on the porch, or in a closet. Even better, purchase some attractive barrels with wheels and tight-fitting lids, and keep them right in your kitchen where they are more accessible. You don't have to worry about any unpleasant odors using this easy composting system. Properly composted earth has a pleasant, woodsy smell.

If more than a few drops of moisture collect under the barrel, the compost is probably too moist. To eliminate any odor that develops, sprinkle a couple of handfuls of lime into the barrel and mix it up with a shovel. Sprinkle some more lime on the top layer, and cover. To avoid this pitfall, cover scraps totally with mats and avoid adding freshly watered mats to the can. Instead, let them dry out until they are moist, but not wet, and cover the surface with a handful of lime.

Composting Instructions Check List

The main points of this easy composting system are reviewed below:

- Obtain 2 barrels and drill holes spaced 2 inches apart all around.

- Place broken-up mats in the bottom of a barrel, followed by vegetable scraps and pulp, a few earthworms, and another layer of broken-up mats to cover. When you have additional mats, repeat the layers, without adding more worms, until the barrel is full. Always re-cover the barrel.

- Let the barrel sit for 2–3 months, at which time your compost will be ready to be mixed with 25 percent peat moss for planting. To speed the composting process, you can stir up the contents of the barrel each week so that the compost will be ready 1 or 2 months later.

If you regularly maintain an outdoor compost pile using a method without animal manures, you may add your mats to it

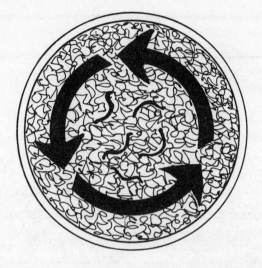

Composting is a way of recycling topsoil.

instead. But during the winter months, you will be better off if you have a ready supply of compost and a few barrels in progress indoors. At the Foundation we send our compost every year or two to our mini-farm in exchange for a fresh supply. The old compost is placed in the gardens, and is reconditioned by the elements. Such a rotation is ideal, as the soil will eventually need to be exposed to the air, rain, and sun, if it is to stay healthy and balanced.

Indoor gardening is a simple, economical, healthful, and ecologically efficient way to supplement your diet. Like sprouting, this endeavor helps you to take responsibility for your own health. Moreover, indoor gardening and proper composting combine to create a system that is virtually self-sufficient—offering you the reward of knowing that you are playing a small but significant role in replenishing the earth's natural resources.

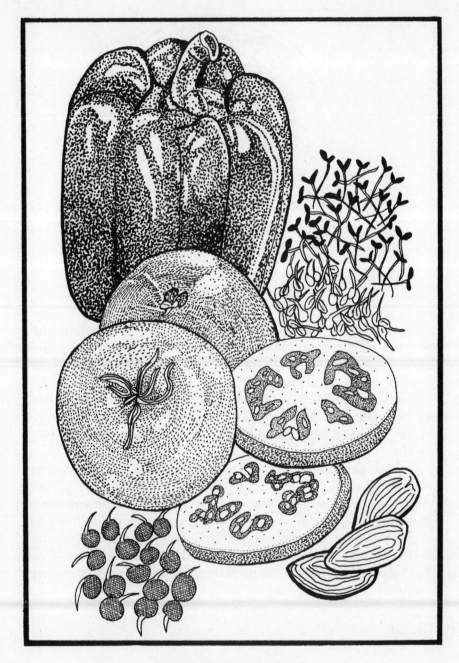

Living Food Ingredients

8

Simple Recipes
with Sprouts

Tall oaks from little acorns grow.

David Everett

The recipes in this chapter show how you can prepare all sorts of delicious meals without cooking. Living foods ingredients include—but are not limited to—sprouts, fresh vegetables, and fresh fruits. To preserve vitamins, minerals, proteins, fats, carbohydrates, enzymes, chlorophyll, and other vital biogenic and bioactive food factors, living foods are never cooked.

The preparation of living foods may involve blending, juicing, grinding, mashing, fermenting, marinating, or drying. Salad ingredients may simply be cut or torn into bite-sized pieces and tossed together; desserts may be chilled or frozen. In these ways, the living foods ingredients are combined to provide an exciting variety of textures, colors, and taste sensations—without compromising the good nutrition that is so important to health.

The first part of this chapter will introduce you to the equipment and methods used in the preparation of living foods recipes containing sprouts. In addition, it contains guidelines that will help you to get the most from your time and energy.

PREPARATION

To prepare these recipes, you may need to make an investment in a few kitchen appliances. A good-quality multi-speed blender will be used often for making beverages, dressings, cheeses, yogurts, soups, and a variety of complete and nourishing meals. A good juicer is essential as well. A blender cannot substitute for a juicer, as a blender will merely liquefy a fruit or vegetable, while a juicer will extract juice and separate it from the pulp. I usually recommend a Champion juicer to my guests at the Ann Wigmore Foundation in Boston, because of its versatility.

Sprouts and greens are delicate, however—too delicate to be juiced in a Champion juicer. At the Ann Wigmore Foundation, we use specially made slow-turning juicers to blend sprouts and greens. For the best results at home, you should obtain one of these.

You will need a couple of sharp knives, a good-sized cutting board, and a vegetable grater to make salads. A fine wire mesh strainer made of stainless steel is important in making blended foods, including juices and other beverages.

Of course, the sprouting supplies described in Chapter 6 (jars, screens, and seeds) are essential. The planting supplies discussed in Chapter 7 (trays and seeds) are recommended as well. To make Rejuvelac, a nutritious beverage that is popular among guests at the Foundation, you will need several additional half-gallon jars with cheesecloth or nylon mesh screens to cover the tops. Made by adding water to sprouted wheatberries, Rejuvelac is called for in some of the sprout recipes.

When you make breads, you will get the best results with a dehydrator. In the Living Food Lifestyle, this useful piece of equipment replaces an oven. It is used for drying vegetable and grain crisps, fresh fruits (when they are inexpensive and in season), pie crusts, and seed loaves as well as breads. However, the recipes in this chapter will also yield satisfactory results if you use your oven at a very low heat—about 105° F. The required drying times may be longer if you use the oven.

You will need plenty of counter space for preparing food. In addition, you may want to clear a space on top of the refrigerator for fermenting seed cheeses and yogurts. When they are left in a warm place, less time is needed to complete the fermentation process. Leave them in glass jars, covered with a clean towel or cheesecloth.

Ingredients to Have on Hand

In order to maintain an abundant supply of sprouts, replenish your stock of seeds, nuts, grains, and beans regularly. Place each variety in its own glass or plastic jar, and make sure that each jar is covered and labeled.

Dried and fresh fruits should also be plentiful in your kitchen. Good-quality dried fruits are available at natural foods stores. Unsulfured fruits, particularly ones that have been sun-dried, are the best kind to buy. Fresh fruits should always be used when they are ripe, and, as much as possible, when they are in season. (You may, however, want to use your dehydrator to dry some fresh fruits, and store them for future use.)

Buy a variety of fresh vegetables frequently. Store the ones that you will not be using immediately (i.e., that same day) in the refrigerator; keep them in covered glass or plastic containers. Refrigeration tends to extract the moisture from foods, leaving them dry and limp unless they are kept covered.

Using These Recipes

For the best possible results, remember that these recipes are intended to provide you with a guide in creating balanced and tasty meals. Don't be afraid to improvise when you are preparing living foods. The exactitudes of baking with white flour and the like are not required. More than anything else, what is needed is common sense. If something seems too dry, add liquid; if it tastes too bland, add flavor with spices or seasonings such as tamari (natural soy sauce). Be creative and adjust the recipes to suit your own tastes.

In many recipes you will find suggestions regarding the number of days that seeds should be sprouted. These suggestions, which appear in parentheses, will help you to match mature sprouts to particular recipes. In general, sprouts used in salads are grown longer and contain more water than those used in loaves or sauces.

To retain maximum freshness, do not wash fresh vegetables until just before you are going to use them. In contrast, unsprouted nuts and seeds should be soaked overnight in pure spring water (unless the recipe specifies otherwise). Soaking, which is in fact the first step in the sprouting process, improves the digestibility and nutritional value of nuts and seeds that are difficult to grow. Dried fruits should also be soaked overnight, but for a different reason; it makes them easier to work with and brings out their flavor.

Measure various amounts of harvested sprouts by gently pressing them into a measuring cup or spoon. Since sprouts are grown and harvested with varying amounts of room around them, this will lend consistency to the recipes.

Each of the recipes in this chapter is designed to serve two people. The bread recipes will generally yield two or more small loaves, about a pound of bread in all. Of course, the amounts can be adjusted as necessary to serve any number of people. Because the freshness of the ingredients is important, however, do not keep leftovers for more than a day or two. Store them in sealable glass or plastic containers in the refrigerator.

RECIPES

Basics

Rejuvelac

½ cup soft pastry wheat
6 cups spring or filtered water

Soak wheatberries in a half-gallon jar, covered with cheesecloth or nylon mesh screening, for 10–15 hours. Drain off water (do not rinse wheatberries) and let wheat sprout for 2 days. After this time, pour water over wheat sprouts (use about three times the amount of wheat sprouts). Cover jar and leave at room temperature for 24 hours. Then pour off liquid Rejuvelac into another jar. Cover and refrigerate; it will keep for several days in this way.

The wheat sprouts can be reused 2 more times to make additional Rejuvelac. Start by pouring more water over sprouts, and proceed as described above.

For fuller-flavored Rejuvelac, you may use the following alternative method. Grind 1-day-old wheat sprouts by lightly blending them with a little water. Pour into a half-gallon jar, add remaining water, cover with a piece of nylon mesh or cheesecloth, and let stand for 3 days. Rejuvelac will be ready to use on the third day. It will have a pleasant smell and slightly lemony flavor when it is ready; it can be stored in a covered jar in the refrigerator for 2–3 days. Ideally, however, Rejuvelac should be served at room temperature.

Basic Seed Cheese

1½ cups sunflower sprouts (1 day)
½ cup sesame sprouts (1 day)
1 cup Rejuvelac

Blend sprouts and Rejuvelac to obtain a thick paste. Pour the mixture into a glass jar, cover with a clean towel or cloth, and leave it for 8–12 hours (the longer it stands the stronger the flavor will be). If you don't have Rejuvelac, you can use a tablespoon of miso (fermented soybean paste) and a cup of water instead. If you use this method, however, the fermentation time may need to be extended to 12–18 hours. After the fermentation time elapses, stick a spoon through the cheese on top and pour off and discard the liquid that has settled at the bottom of the jar. Try making this cheese with sprouted almonds. Combinations of sprouted almonds, sunflower sprouts, and sesame sprouts are also very flavorful. Store extra cheese in the refrigerator; covered tightly, it will keep for 5 days.

Basic Seed Yogurt
---

1 cup sunflower sprouts (1 day)
½ cup sesame sprouts (1 day)
2 cups Rejuvelac

Blend sprouts and Rejuvelac to a smooth consistency. Pour the mixture into a glass jar, cover with a clean towel or cloth, and let it stand for 8–12 hours. Stir the yogurt before use. Also try making Almond Yogurt, using 2 cups of almond sprouts in place of the sunflower and sesame. Store unused yogurt in the refrigerator; like seed cheese, it will keep for several days if covered tightly.

Beverages

Milks

Almond Milk

½ cup almond sprouts (1 day)
½ cup pine nuts, soaked six hours
4 cups spring or filtered water

Place almond sprouts, pine nuts, and water in blender and blend on high speed for 2 minutes. Strain out pulp.

Carob Milk
---

4 cups Almond *or* Wheat Milk
½ cup pitted dates, soaked
2 tablespoons carob powder

Blend ingredients for 2 minutes at high speed.

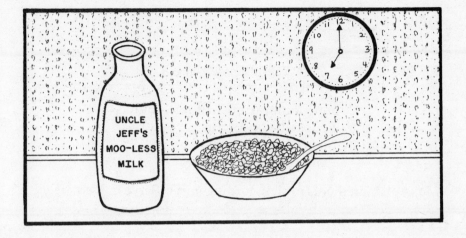

Sesame Milkshake

---

1 cup sesame sprouts (1 day)
4 cups spring or filtered water
1 medium banana
1 tablespoon maple syrup

Blend sesame sprouts with water at high speed for 3 minutes.
Strain through a fine wire mesh strainer to remove pulp, and
return liquid to blender. Add banana and maple syrup, blend
at medium speed for 2 minutes, and serve chilled.

Wheat Milk

---

1 cup wheat sprouts (2 days)
4–6 cups spring or filtered water
½ cup raisins, soaked

Blend wheat sprouts with water for 2 minutes at high speed.
Strain through a fine wire mesh strainer, discarding pulp and
returning liquid to blender. Add raisins; blend and strain as
before.

Juices

Carrot-Sprout Juice
---

6 medium carrots, cut into chunks
2 cups alfalfa sprouts
1 cup mung sprouts
1 cup buckwheat greens

Juice all ingredients in slow-turning juicer. Serve immediately.

Green Drink
---

2 cups alfalfa sprouts
2 cups buckwheat greens
2 cups sunflower greens
½ cup mung sprouts
1 medium carrot, cut into chunks
1 celery stalk
½ medium cucumber
4 parsley sprigs

Juice all ingredients in slow-turning juicer.

Pine-Alfa Juice

½ pineapple
1½ cups alfalfa sprouts
1 mint sprig (optional)

Peel pineapple and juice in high-speed juicer. Blend with other ingredients at high speed for 1 minute, and serve chilled.

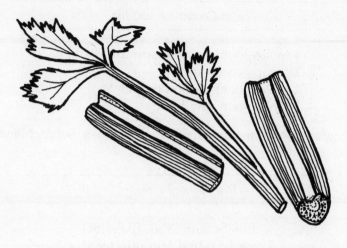

Sweet and Spicy

---

2 cups alfalfa sprouts
½ cup cabbage sprouts
¼ cup radish sprouts
1 medium cucumber
1 sweet red pepper, cut into chunks
1 medium carrot, cut into chunks

Juice all ingredients in slow-turning juicer.

Smoothies

Blueberry Smoothie

---

4 cups Almond Milk (page 80)
1 cup blueberries
1 medium banana

Blend ingredients at medium speed for 2 minutes. Serve chilled.

Carob-Coconut Smoothie
---

4 tablespoons sesame sprouts (1 day)
2½ cups coconut milk
2 tablespoons carob powder
1 tablespoon raw honey

Blend ingredients at medium speed for 2 minutes. Serve chilled.

Peaches and Cream
---

4 cups Sesame Milk (page 81)
1 peach, pitted and quartered
1 tablespoon vanilla

Blend ingredients at medium speed for 2 minutes. Serve chilled.

Strawberry Whirl
---

2 cups Almond Milk (page 80)
2 cups Sesame Milk (page 81)
1 cup strawberries, trimmed
1 tablespoon maple syrup

Blend all ingredients.

Breakfast Dishes

Nutty Cereal
---

1 cup sunflower sprouts (2 days)
1 cup almond sprouts (1–2 days)
½ cup raisins, soaked
2 cups spring or filtered water,
    Rejuvelac (page 78), *or* apple juice

Blend ingredients for 1 minute at medium speed.

Pine-Nut Crunch Cereal

---

1 cup wheat sprouts (2–3 days)
½ cup sesame sprouts (1 day)
½ cup rye sprouts (2 days)
1 cup pine nuts, soaked 6 hours
1 medium banana, sliced

Mix ingredients in a bowl. Serve with Almond Milk (page 80).

Sprouted Wheat-Prune Cereal

---

8 pitted prunes
3 cups wheat sprouts (2–3 days)
½ medium apple
spring or filtered water

Soak prunes in 1 cup of water overnight. Blend prunes and water from soaking them with other ingredients, adding more water as needed to obtain a soup-like consistency. For variety, try making this cereal with figs instead of prunes.

Breads

Basic Bread

4–6 cups wheat *and/or* rye sprouts (1 day)
1 teaspoon caraway seeds

Run sprouts through a grinder, a slow-turning juicer with the end screw detached, or a Champion juicer, or blend in a food processor with a little water. The Champion juicer with the homogenizing blank inserted makes a fine smooth dough. Be sure to feed the sprouts into the juicer slowly, so that the motor will not overheat. Mix in the caraway seeds. Press the dough into a small, flat, wafer-like loaf. Place it on an oiled cookie sheet or on a dryer rack, and dry it in a dehydrator or in a warm oven set at 105° F. The bread will take from 12 to 20 hours to become crisp.

Banana Grain Crisps
---

3 cups wheat sprouts (1 day)
2½ cups Rejuvelac (page 78) *or*
    spring or filtered water
1 large banana
½ teaspoon cinnamon

Blend sprouted grain with liquid to obtain a smooth batter. Quickly blend in banana and cinnamon. Pour onto oiled cookie sheets and dry in dehydrator or low-heat oven (105° F) for about 18 hours or until crisp. For variety, try making grain crisps with ½ cup of soaked raisins instead of bananas.

Chick Pea Wheat Bread
---

2 cups chick pea sprouts (2 days)
2 cups wheat sprouts (1 day)
1 teaspoon cumin
1 teaspoon tamari

Grind chick pea and wheat sprouts to make dough as described in Basic Bread recipe. Mix in seasonings and form into flat loaves. Dry in dehydrator or low-heat oven (105° F) for about 18 hours or until crisp.

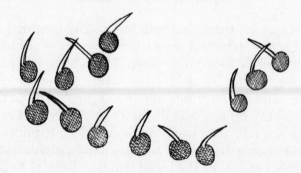

Grain Crisps
---

3 cups wheat *or* rye sprouts (1 day)
2½ cups Rejuvelac (page 78) *or*
  spring or filtered water
caraway seeds, dried onion, or other
  seasonings (optional)

Blend all ingredients at high speed until smooth. Pour batter ¼ inch thick onto oiled cookie sheet. Dry in dehydrator or low-heat oven (105° F) until crisp; this will take approximately 18 hours. Break into small pieces when dry.

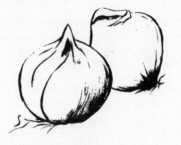

Pizza Bread
---

4 cups wheat sprouts (1 day)
½ large red pepper, thinly sliced
½ tomato, chopped
½ small onion, thinly sliced
¼ cup black olives, thinly sliced
2 garlic cloves, pressed
½ teaspoon Italian seasoning mix

Grind wheat in grinder or Champion juicer, or blend in food processor with a little water, as described in Basic Bread recipe. Shape dough into flat, ½-inch-thick loaves on a cookie sheet. Dry in dehydrator or low-heat oven (105° F) for 12 hours or until almost crisp. Top with other ingredients and dry for another 6–8 hours, or until topping and crust are both dry.

Sourdough Rye Bread
---

3 cups rye sprouts (1 day)
1 cup wheat sprouts
1 teaspoon caraway seeds

Grind sprouts in a grinder or juicer, or blend in a food processor with a little water, as described in the recipe for Basic Bread. Place dough in a bowl and mix in caraway seeds. Cover with a clean towel or cloth and leave overnight to sour. Shape dough into flat loaves ½ inch thick; dry in a dehydrator, in an oven, or in the sun until crisp.

Soups

Carrot Soup
---

6 medium carrots
½ beet
½ medium cucumber
½ cup alfalfa sprouts

Juice carrots and beet in high-speed juicer. Blend with cucumbers and sprouts at high speed for 2 minutes. Serve with Sourdough Rye Bread (above).

Cream of Cauliflower Soup

1½ cups cauliflower flowerets
    (⅓ medium head)
1 cup lentil sprouts (3 days)
1 cup pine nuts, soaked 6 hours
1 parsley sprig
½ teaspoon cumin
2–3 cups spring or filtered water

Blend first five ingredients at high speed, adding water until a smooth but thick consistency is reached. Serve with Basic Bread (page 85).

Cream of Spinach Soup

3 cups spinach
½ cup Basic Seed Yogurt (page 80)
    or ½ large avocado
½ medium tomato
1 scallion
2 cups spring or filtered water
1 tablespoon tamari
10 medium mushrooms, thinly sliced

Blend all ingredients except mushrooms at high speed until smooth. Garnish individual servings with thinly sliced mushrooms.

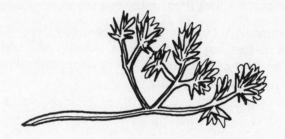

Original Gazpacho

3 medium tomatoes
1 cup spring or filtered water
1 cup alfalfa sprouts
½ medium cucumber
2 celery stalk tops
½ scallion
½ garlic clove
1 parsley sprig
¼ teaspoon Italian seasoning mix
4 tablespoons lemon juice
1 pinch cayenne pepper (optional)

First blend tomatoes and water at medium speed for 1 minute; then blend in other ingredients. Serve with lentil sprouts and Pizza Bread (page 87).

Sprout Soup
---

1 cup buckwheat greens
1 cup sunflower greens
1 cup alfalfa sprouts
1 cup mung sprouts
1 celery stalk
1 medium carrot, cut into chunks
½ medium cucumber, quartered
¼ cup parsley
⅛ cup scallions, finely chopped
½ sweet red pepper, diced
½ avocado, cubed
1 tablespoon tamari

Juice all ingredients except for scallions, red pepper, and avocado in slow-turning juicer. Mix in tamari, add scallions and avocado, and serve with a side dish of chopped red pepper and some sprouted wheat bread.

Salads

Sprout and Vegetable Salads

Lentil Sea Salad
---

2 cups lentil sprouts (3 days)
¼ cup dulse sea vegetable (dry), chopped
¼ cup scallions, chopped
¼ tomato *or* sweet red pepper, chopped
¼ celery stalk, chopped
¼ medium avocado, chopped
1 teaspoon lemon juice
1 teaspoon tamari

Mix vegetables and avocado in a salad bowl. Combine lemon juice and tamari and pour over salad.

Marinated Sprouts and Vegetables
---

1 cup mung sprouts
½ cup adzuki sprouts
½ cup cabbage sprouts
½ sweet red pepper, thinly sliced
15 snow pea pods, quartered
4 medium stalks Chinese cabbage, chopped
½ celery stalk, cut into matchsticks
2 garlic cloves, pressed
¼ cup scallions, chopped
¼ cup tamari
3 tablespoons lemon juice
spring or filtered water

Marinate sprouts and vegetables for 2–4 hours in a mixture of tamari, lemon juice, and a little water. Stir occasionally so that all the vegetables are marinated. Serve on a bed of lettuce and top with avocado cubes.

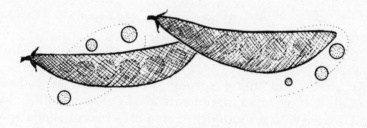

Spinach Salad
---

4 cups spinach
1 cup mung sprouts
8 medium mushrooms, thinly sliced
½ small red onion, thinly sliced
½ cup Grain Crisps (page 87),
    broken into croutons

Tear spinach into medium-sized pieces. Toss with other ingredients in a salad bowl. Serve with lemon juice or Creamy Lemon Dressing (page 95).

Sprout Garden Salad
---

4 large leaves romaine lettuce
1 cup alfalfa sprouts
1 cup buckwheat greens
½ cup lentil sprouts (3 days)
1 tomato, cubed
½ celery stalk, chopped
½ sweet red pepper, chopped

Tear lettuce into medium-sized pieces. Toss with other ingredients in a salad bowl. Serve with lemon juice or Russian Dressing (page 96).

Stuffed Salad
---

2 cups alfalfa sprouts
1 cup mung sprouts
1 tomato, diced
½ medium avocado, chopped
1 tablespoon tamari
6 outer leaves romaine lettuce

Mix alfalfa and mung sprouts with tomato, avocado, and tamari. Roll up salad ingredients inside romaine lettuce leaves and secure with a toothpick. Serve on a bed of alfalfa sprouts with some sauerkraut on the side.

Watercress Salad
---

1 cup alfalfa sprouts
1 small bunch watercress, chopped
½ celery stalk, finely chopped
½ medium avocado, cubed
1 tablespoon lemon juice

Toss salad ingredients and serve with Spring Green Dressing (page 96).

Winter Sprout Salad

½ cup wheat sprouts (3 days)
½ cup lentil sprouts (3 days)
½ cup alfalfa sprouts
½ cup buckwheat greens
½ cup sunflower greens
½ medium carrot, finely grated
¼ cup red onion, thinly sliced

Toss all ingredients in a salad bowl. Serve with Parsley-Garlic Dressing (page 95).

Sprout and Fruit Salads

Blueberries and Cream

½ cup pine nuts, soaked 6 hours
½ cup spring or filtered water
1 tablespoon maple syrup
3 pints blueberries

Blend pine nuts, water, and maple syrup at high speed for 2 minutes. Pour over individual servings of fresh blueberries.

Citrus Almond Salad
---

1 medium orange, peeled and chopped
½ pink grapefruit, peeled and chopped
10 medium strawberries, sliced
½ cup orange juice
¼ cup almond sprouts

Mix orange, grapefruit, and strawberries. Blend orange juice with sprouted almonds for 2 minutes at high speed. Pour over salad ingredients.

Dried Fruit Salad
---

4 dried pitted apricots, chopped
4 dried figs, chopped
1 dried pear (2 halves), chopped
8 slices dried apple, chopped
½ cup almond sprouts (1 day), chopped
¼ cup sesame sprouts (1 day)
spring or filtered water

Soak dried fruits in water overnight. Pour off water and re-serve. Chop dried fruits and mix them with almond sprouts. Blend ¼ cup of the reserved water with sesame sprouts for 2 minutes at high speed, and pour over salad as a dressing.

Prune-Apple Salad

½ cup almond sprouts, chopped
2 medium apples, peeled and chopped
10 pitted prunes, soaked and chopped
¼ cup grated coconut

Mix almond sprouts, apples, and prunes. Sprinkle grated coconut on top.

Tropical Salad
---

1 medium mango, peeled and cubed
½ papaya, peeled and cubed
1 medium banana, sliced
¼ cup pine nuts, soaked 6 hours
½ cup orange juice

Mix fruits. Blend pine nuts with orange juice at high speed for 2 minutes and pour over salad.

Sprout and Vegetable Salad Dressings

Carrot Dressing
---

4 medium carrots
⅛ beet
½ cup walnuts, soaked 6 hours
1 tablespoon tamari

Juice carrots and beet in high-speed juicer. Blend juice with other ingredients at high speed until smooth.

Creamy Lemon Dressing

¼ cup pine nuts, soaked 6 hours
¼ cup spring or filtered water
2 tablespoons lemon juice
½ teaspoon raw honey

Blend ingredients at high speed for 2 minutes, until creamy For variety, try using sesame sprouts instead of pine nuts.

Parsley-Garlic Dressing

½ cup sunflower sprouts (1 day)
⅛ cup parsley
¼ garlic clove
⅔ cup spring or filtered water
2 tablespoons lemon juice
1 teaspoon tamari

Blend ingredients at high speed to obtain a creamy consistency.

Russian Dressing

½ cup sprouted pumpkin seeds (1 day)
¼ beet
⅛ scallion
⅔ cup spring or filtered water
1 teaspoon tamari

Blend all ingredients at high speed for 2 minutes. Serve with Sprout Garden Salad (page 92).

Spicy Radish Dressing

¼ cup alfalfa sprouts
¼ cup radish sprouts
¼ tomato, cut into chunks
¼ sweet red pepper, cut in half
1 pinch cayenne pepper
⅓ cup spring or filtered water
1 teaspoon tamari

Blend all ingredients at high speed for 2 minutes.

Spring Green Dressing

¼ cup spinach
¼ cup alfalfa sprouts
¼ tomato, cut into chunks
¼ medium avocado, cubed
¼ scallion
⅔ cup spring or filtered water
1 tablespoon tamari

Blend ingredients at high speed for 2 minutes.

Entrees

Chick Pea Hummus
---

    2 cups chick pea sprouts (2 days)
    ½ cup sesame sprouts (1 day)
    ¼ celery stalk, diced
    1 garlic clove, pressed
    1½ cups spring or filtered water
    2 tablespoons lemon juice
    2 teaspoons tamari

Grind, blend, or food-process chick pea and sesame sprouts until smooth. Add other ingredients and mix well.

Lentil Croquettes
---

    3 cups lentil sprouts (3 days)
    1 large carrot, finely grated
    1 scallion, minced
    1½ cups Basic Seed Cheese (page 79)
    ¼ teaspoon cumin

Grind lentil sprouts in food processor; remove and mix with vegetables and seed cheese. Mix in spices, and roll mixture into croquettes (the amounts listed above will make about 12). Serve croquettes on a bed of lettuce and tomato.

Spicy Guacamole
---

    3 medium avocados
    ¼ cup radish sprouts
    2 tablespoons lemon juice
    1 garlic clove, pressed

Mash avocados with fork and mix with other ingredients. Serve with your favorite salad.

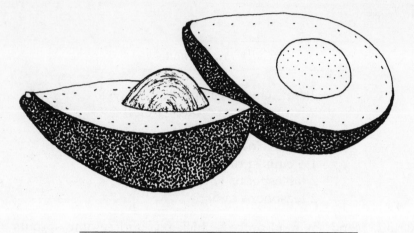

Sprout Loaf
---

1 cup coarsely ground almond sprouts
  (almond meal)
½ cup mung sprouts
½ cup alfalfa sprouts
½ cup cabbage sprouts
¼ sweet red pepper, chopped
¼ celery stalk, chopped
1 tablespoon tamari
spring or filtered water

Mix ingredients with enough water to bind into a loaf. Serve
surrounded with lettuce and sliced vegetables.

Stuffed Peppers
---

1 cup alfalfa sprouts
1 cup lentil sprouts
½ medium avocado, mashed
1 teaspoon tamari
4 green or sweet red peppers, hollowed out

Mix sprouts, avocado, tamari, and lemon juice together in a
bowl. Stuff mixture into hollowed-out peppers and serve on a
bed of alfalfa sprouts.

Desserts

Apple Strudel

Crust:

¼ cup walnuts, soaked 6 hours
12 medium pitted dates, mashed

Filling:

1 apple, minced
¼ cup raisins, soaked
¼ cup walnuts, soaked 6 hours
½ teaspoon cinnamon
2 tablespoons maple syrup
1 teaspoon lemon juice

Grind walnuts for crust and filling in a nut mill, food processor, or blender. Mix filling ingredients well and set aside. To make crust, mix ingredients together well with hands. Roll out crust between two sheets of waxed paper to a thickness of ¼ inch, and cut it into rectangles about 5″ × 12″. Spread filling evenly across each rectangle, making sure that mixture extends to edges of dough. Roll each piece up to create strudel, slice into 2-inch pieces, and dust with powdered almond meal.

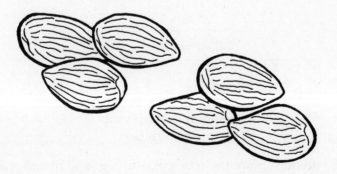

Banana Cream Pie

Crust:

½ cup almond sprouts
½ cup wheat germ
1 banana
1 tablespoon raw honey
1 teaspoon olive oil

Filling:

4 bananas
1 ripe avocado, pitted
2 teaspoons pineapple juice
½ teaspoon vanilla

Cream Topping:

½ cup pine nuts, soaked 6 hours
½ cup spring or filtered water
1 tablespoon maple syrup

To make crust, grind almonds and mix with other ingredients. Press into an oiled pie plate. Mash filling ingredients together with a fork and fill pie shell. Blend pine nuts, water, and maple syrup to make cream topping and pour over pie. Sprinkle shredded coconut on top. Serve chilled.

Banana-Nut Ice Cream

---

4 bananas
½ cup pine nuts, soaked 6 hours
1 teaspoon maple syrup
¼ teaspoon vanilla

Peel bananas, place them in a plastic bag, and freeze overnight. Frozen bananas will keep for 2 weeks in the freezer. Run bananas and pine nuts through a Champion juicer with homogenization blank in place (a blender or food processor may be used instead). The consistency should be similar to that of soft ice cream. Stir in vanilla and maple syrup. Banana-Nut Ice Cream may be served right away or re-frozen for up to 30 minutes before it is served.

Carob Pudding

½ cup almond sprouts
1½ cups spring or filtered water
12 medium pitted dates
5 teaspoons carob powder
1 tablespoon raw honey

Blend almond sprouts with water. Add other ingredients and blend at high speed until smooth.

Dried Fruit Candy
---

6 medium pitted dates
½ cup raisins
6 medium dried figs
4 tablespoons spring or filtered water
2 tablespoons maple syrup
1 cup coarsely ground sunflower
   sprouts (meal)

Grind dried fruits together in slow-turning juicer, nut mill, or food processor. Roll fruit mixture into 1-inch balls and set aside. Mix water and maple syrup in a shallow bowl. Dip dried fruit balls in liquid and roll in sprouted sunflower meal to coat.

Sprouted Wheat Treats
---

1 cup wheat sprouts (2 days)
¼ cup almond sprouts
12 pitted dates
¾ cup shredded coconut
¼ cup sesame seeds, finely ground
1 tablespoon orange juice
1 teaspoon lemon rind, grated

Grind sprouts, dates, and coconut in slow-turning juicer, nut mill, or food processor. Mix in other ingredients. Shape Sprouted Wheat Treats as desired and chill before serving.

9

Sprouts for Travel and for Your Pets

And God said, Behold, I have given you every herb bearing seed, which is upon the face of all the earth, and every tree, in the which is the fruit of a tree yielding seed; to you it shall be for meat.

Gen. 1:29

As fresh sprouts are a key element in any truly healthful diet, it is important that they be readily available to you—and your pets—wherever you go. In this chapter, I will share a few tips that will show you how growing sprouts "on the road" can be easy and lots of fun. With the stresses that travel often imposes, good-quality nutrition is essential. Your pets also can benefit from the vitamins, minerals, enzymes, and energy in sprouts. In the second part of this chapter, I will present a few simple guidelines for feeding sprouts to household pets.

TRAVELING WITH SPROUTS

The most convenient way to travel with sprouts is to grow some before you go to take along with you, and to start some on the way. As I mentioned in Chapter 6, the easiest way to grow sprouts while you're traveling is in sprout bags. They are convenient wherever and whenever you go, and no matter how you travel. When you are in transit, the sprout bags may be temporarily sealed in plastic bags and stored with your luggage.

Take out the sprout bags two or three times a day, rinse the sprouts in cool water, and drain off the excess water. Either hang up the sprout bags or put them back in the plastic. At all times, handle the sprouts as gently as possible, and avoid crushing them. Also bear in mind that extended exposure to either high heat or direct sunlight will damage the sprouts. When properly cared for, however, they will mature in the same amount of time as they would at home.

Sprouting in bags is ideal for camping, boating, hiking, and bike touring. A plastic bag with a sprout bag inside it can be strapped on the outside of a backpack, or placed in a side pocket. It is good to keep the sprouts handy, because they provide the essential ingredients and ready energy that you need for vigorous out-of-doors activities.

If you are traveling by car, you may want to bring along a few jars for sprouting and some trays for growing greens. As long as you remember that the interior of a car can heat up very quickly, and take care not to leave the young plants in direct sunlight for an extended period of time, they will probably do quite well. If you also bring an insulated cooler filled with harvested sprouts, fresh vegetables, fruits, live food salad dressings, and other supplies, you will have a reliable source of nutritious food close at hand, with a minimum of fuss.

When I travel, I take a variety of seeds and already prepared sprouts with me. On my frequent airplane trips, other passengers watch enviously as I toss together a sprout salad in a bowl that I bring along. With fresh sprouts, a few slices of tomato, and a little home-made dressing, I am all set to dine like royalty. My experience shows that there is no need for anyone to suffer through an unpalatable airline meal that causes indigestion and exhaustion after the plane lands. You can take sprouts everywhere, and you will be healthier and happier for doing so.

SPROUTS FOR YOUR PETS

For years I have fed sprouted seeds and beans to my dogs and cats, because these animals suffer unnecessarily from many "human" ailments. Apart from humans, they are the only creatures on earth who eat their food cooked. Yet it is clear that they crave and need fresh foods. They often insist upon eating grass and green weeds, even though these frequently cause coughing or gagging.

With the addition of sprouts and other live foods to their diet, all kinds of pets can avoid suffering and illness throughout life. In many cases, they are even able to control and reverse illnesses that are already in progress.

Modern pets, like modern people, need sprouts, but getting animals to understand this can be frustrating at times! Nevertheless, my pets have always enjoyed good health and had glossy coats, improved vision, and a sweet disposition because of sprouts. If you are patient, you can have the same success in getting the most nutrition out of sprouts for your pets, and in getting them to enjoy eating sprouts.

Begin by adding sprouts and raw vegetables to your pet's diet slowly. Since dogs and cats are notorious for bolting their food, it's important for you to chop sprouts and vegetables into fine pieces before mixing about four tablespoons (or more) of them in with the canned or dried food your pet usually eats. Don't give up in the beginning if your pet takes a bite of food and walks away uninterested. It may not be hungry, or it may be hesitant about trying food with an unfamiliar flavor and aroma. Just leave the bowl of food accessible, and your pet will return when it gets hungry.

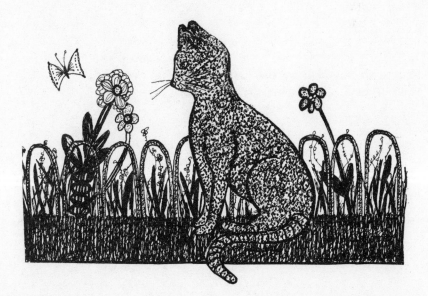

With especially finicky animals, you may need to start out using smaller amounts of the chopped sprouts. Never force these healthful ingredients on an animal—in a show of stubbornness, it could refuse to eat any of its food. And in most cases, a nagging, half-hungry, half-angry pet can outlast a pet owner, who gets frustrated and gives in easily. To enhance your pet's health, increase the amount of sprouts in its food slowly.

In a few weeks, your pet may be willing to eat up to one-half cup of sprouts per day (maybe more, depending on its size and appetite). This is enough to make up for the nutritional deficiencies in modern pet food, and your pet will hardly put up a fuss about it.

When the animals who depend on you for food, shelter, and affection are healthier (because they eat sprouts), they'll be happier—and you will be, too.

Epilogue

Sprouts: Food for a New Generation

I've seed de first and de last. . . . I seed de beginning, en now I sees the endin.

William Faulkner

Over the years the popularity of sprouting has grown steadily, and today it seems that sprouts are here to stay. And as more people become aware of the nutritional and economic value of sprouts, they respond in the same way as so many others who have attended one of my lectures—by asking when they can begin growing and using sprouts.

The answer, of course, is now. Just a few days from now, you and your family can be enjoying the flavor and health benefits of sprouts. Given the availability of automatic growers and mail order seed sources, sprouting is accessible to anybody, regardless of his or her schedule or lifestyle. It is my hope that the information contained in this book will eliminate any potential confusion or problems you may have with the actual growing of sprouts.

Since the late 1950s I have taught thousands of people how to grow their own food at home. Those who have visited the Ann Wigmore Foundation in Boston have often been amazed and surprised to see how much food one person can actually grow—enough to feed twenty people at any given time. And how little time it takes to do so! Yet, growing a portion of your own fresh live foods at home is one of the most important things you can do. In this way you will be controlling your diet—and your health. The advantages to having control over your food supply are obvious, as cancer, heart disease, and other degenerative illnesses are linked to poor eating habits.

Living foods—sprouts, greens, wheatgrass, fresh vegetables, and fresh fruits—are the key to a healthy body and a longer, more satisfying life. They can protect us from the ravages of illness by strengthening our immunity. In addition, living foods help our overall metabolism, keeping us clean and balanced inside. Biological mechanisms like the human body cannot thrive, or even survive, on synthetic processed foods and chemicals, which make up more than half of the present diet in the Western World. The absence of live foods in the typical modern diet spells doom for many people, but you need not be one of them.

At present, there is a well-grounded movement towards "natural" foods and body care products in the United States. And though this shift in consciousness is rather slow, it is definitely heading in the right direction. Many prominent nutritionists, political leaders, entertainers, and physicians are leading the way by espousing (and living) a more natural lifestyle. Yet, despite the fact that many so-called health foods are natural products, they are not infused with life energies. Years of work in the health field have taught me that foods *must* be eaten uncooked for us to gain their full benefits. Until nutritionists and medical scientists, as a group, recognize the importance of living (biogenic and bioactive) foods, our society is bound to be plagued by the thousands of health problems we suffer from today.

The problems of world hunger and malnutrition will not be solved with synthetic processed foods, dried milk powder, and meat. The very production of meat, milk, and other animal foods is in large part responsible for these problems. It requires about thirty times more land and energy (oil, gas, electricity, and so on) to produce a pound of meat or cheese than it does to produce one pound of sprouts.

Another reason that meat and milk are not effective in combating world hunger is that they are poor sources of energy-producing carbohydrates. Every day, the body needs more carbohydrates for energy than proteins and fats for building (growth and repair). The day is not far off when developing nations will make feeding their people a top priority. And when that day comes, sprouts will be a logical choice for accomplishing this important task. In most cases, surplus seeds and beans for sprouting are available; it is merely information about using them in their sprouted form that is missing.

No amount of surgery, pills, therapy, or money can keep us well. Only a desire and willingness to learn more about nature, and to embrace her laws, can do so. This means that we must eat foods such as sprouts, greens, wheatgrass, fruits, and vegetables, with all of their vital nutrients intact—in their natural, living state. Sprouts are at the very top of this list of vital foods.

Throughout this book, I have discussed some of the ways in which sprouts can play a significant role in nourishing and protecting the health of people everywhere. Even more so than the other living foods, sprouts have the potential to start each and every one of us on the way towards independence in matters of diet and health. Growing and eating them can help us to assume self-responsibility for the single most important resource we own—the human body and its health. Won't you join me (and thousands of other people around the world) today, in growing and eating an abundance of fresh, life-giving sprouts?

For more information regarding sprouting
or the Ann Wigmore Institute, please contact:

Ann Wigmore Institute
P.O. Box 429
Rincon, PR 00677
(787) 868-6307 phone
(787) 868-2430 fax

Ann Wigmore Foundation
P.O. Box 399
San Fidel, NM 87049
(505) 552-0595

Index